Prioritization & Delegation

for Nursing Students

A Complete Workbook

Dr. David P. Zapencki, DNP, MSN/Ed, CNE, CCRN

Professional Development Publishing

Published by Professional Development Publishing.

ISBN 978-1-971135-04-5 (Paperback)
ISBN 978-1-971135-05-2 (Ebook)

Table of Contents

[Update field to generate TOC]

Preface

Why This Workbook?

Every experienced nurse can recall a moment early in their career when they felt completely overwhelmed. Multiple patients needed attention simultaneously. Tasks competed for time that seemed impossibly short. The question "What do I do first?" felt paralyzing rather than answerable.

If you are a nursing student or new graduate facing similar moments, know this: you are not alone, and these feelings do not reflect a personal failing. Prioritization and delegation are among the most challenging skills in nursing—and among the most important. They are skills that develop over time, with practice, guidance, and deliberate effort.

This workbook exists because I believe that development does not have to happen only through trial and error at the bedside. While nothing replaces clinical experience, structured learning can accelerate your growth and build confidence before you face high-stakes situations with real patients. The frameworks, principles, and practice scenarios in these pages are designed to give you mental tools you can rely on when the pressure is high and the decisions are consequential.

The Critical Nature of These Skills

Prioritization and delegation are not merely academic topics to master for an examination. They are, quite literally, matters of life and death.

Research consistently demonstrates that a significant proportion of preventable patient deaths are preceded by warning signs that were missed or not acted upon in time. Nurses who can rapidly identify deteriorating patients, allocate their attention appropriately, and mobilize team resources effectively are nurses who save lives. Conversely, nurses who become mired in low-priority tasks while critical needs go unaddressed contribute to the tragic phenomenon known as "failure to rescue."

Beyond patient safety, these skills affect your own well-being. Nurses who struggle with prioritization experience higher rates of burnout, anxiety, and job dissatisfaction. They stay late, skip breaks, and carry the weight of feeling perpetually behind. In contrast, nurses who develop strong prioritization and delegation abilities report greater confidence, better work-life balance, and longer, more fulfilling careers.

The stakes are high. But so is your capacity to learn.

How This Workbook Is Organized

This workbook follows a deliberate progression from foundational concepts to integrated application:

Chapters 1 and 2 establish the foundations of prioritization. You will learn what prioritization means in nursing practice, why it matters for patient safety, and how clinical judgment develops over time. You will also learn the major frameworks—ABCs, Maslow's Hierarchy of Needs, acute versus chronic, and actual versus potential—that guide priority-setting in different clinical contexts.

Chapters 3 and 4 introduce the principles of delegation. You will learn the Five Rights of Delegation, understand the legal and professional accountability that accompanies delegation decisions, and develop a clear understanding of scope of practice for registered nurses, licensed practical nurses, and unlicensed assistive personnel.

Chapters 5 and 6 address the practical aspects of working with teams. You will learn how to make safe patient assignments, how to communicate effectively when delegating, how to select appropriate levels of supervision, and how to handle situations when things do not go as planned.

Chapter 7 brings everything together through clinical application. You will learn systematic approaches like the PRIOD method, work through realistic case studies, and develop strategies for managing time and avoiding common pitfalls.

Chapter 8 provides comprehensive practice with fifty NCLEX-style questions that integrate concepts from all previous chapters, preparing you for both the licensure examination and real-world clinical practice.

Each chapter includes learning objectives, detailed content with examples, and practice problems with thorough rationales. The Answer Key at the end of the workbook provides not just correct answers but explanations of why each answer is right and why the alternatives are wrong.

How to Use This Workbook

I encourage you to approach this workbook actively rather than passively. Do not simply read the content—engage with it.

Work through the practice problems honestly. Cover the answers and attempt each question before checking your response. When you get a question wrong, do not simply note the correct answer and move on. Read the rationale carefully. Understand why the correct answer is correct and why your chosen answer was not the best option. This reflective practice builds deeper understanding than passive reading ever could.

Connect the content to your clinical experiences. As you encounter patients in clinical rotations, ask yourself: Which framework applies here? What would I delegate? How would I communicate this? The workbook provides the concepts; clinical practice provides the context. Together, they build competence.

Return to earlier chapters as needed. Learning is not always linear. If you find yourself struggling with delegation scenarios in Chapter 6, you may benefit from reviewing the Five Rights in Chapter 3 or the scope of practice content in Chapter 4. Use the workbook as a reference, not just a one-time read.

Practice with others when possible. Discussing clinical scenarios with classmates or colleagues deepens understanding. You will learn from their perspectives, and teaching concepts to others reinforces your own mastery.

A Note on Clinical Judgment

Throughout this workbook, you will encounter the phrase "clinical judgment" repeatedly. Clinical judgment is the ability to make sound decisions in complex, uncertain situations—and it is the heart of nursing practice.

The NCSBN Clinical Judgment Measurement Model, which underlies the Next Generation NCLEX, describes clinical judgment as a cycle: recognizing cues, analyzing their meaning, prioritizing hypotheses, generating solutions, taking action, and evaluating outcomes. This model appears throughout the workbook because it reflects how expert nurses actually think.

As a student, you are building clinical judgment with every patient encounter, every simulation, and every practice problem you complete. The frameworks in this workbook are not meant to replace clinical judgment but to support its development. They provide structure when experience is limited and scaffolding while intuition develops.

Trust the process. With time and practice, what now requires conscious, step-by-step reasoning will become more automatic. The competent nurse becomes proficient; the proficient nurse becomes expert. This workbook is one step on that journey.

Acknowledgments

No educational resource is created in isolation. I am grateful to the colleagues, students, and mentors who have shaped my understanding of nursing education over the years. I am particularly indebted to the nursing students who have shared their struggles and successes with prioritization and delegation—their experiences directly informed the content and examples in these pages.

I also acknowledge the foundational work of Patricia Benner, whose research on novice-to-expert development continues to illuminate how nurses grow; Abraham Maslow, whose hierarchy of needs provides an enduring framework for understanding human priorities; and the National Council of State Boards of Nursing, whose work on delegation guidelines and clinical judgment has advanced nursing practice and education.

Finally, I thank you, the reader, for your commitment to learning. Nursing is challenging, demanding, and sometimes overwhelming—but it is also meaningful, rewarding, and profoundly important. The skills you develop through this workbook will serve your patients, your profession, and your own well-being for years to come.

Welcome to the journey.

Dr. David P. Zapencki, DNP, MSN/Ed, CNE, CCRN

CHAPTER 1

Foundations of Prioritization

1.1 Learning Objectives

By the end of this chapter, you will be able to:

- Define prioritization in the context of nursing practice
- Explain the relationship between prioritization and patient safety
- Describe how clinical judgment informs priority-setting
- Identify how prioritization is tested on the NCLEX-RN

1.2 What Is Prioritization?

Prioritization is the process of determining which patient needs require immediate attention and which can safely wait. It sounds simple enough, but in practice, prioritization is one of the most challenging skills a nurse must develop. Every shift, you will face competing demands: multiple patients, various tasks, unexpected changes, and limited time. Your ability to sort through these demands and address the most critical needs first can mean the difference between a good outcome and a devastating one.

A Continuous Process

One of the most important things to understand about prioritization is that it never stops. You do not prioritize once at the beginning of your shift and then follow a fixed plan. Patient conditions change—sometimes gradually, sometimes in an instant. A patient who was stable an hour ago may now be showing signs of respiratory distress. The admission you were expecting gets delayed, but a different patient suddenly spikes a fever.

Effective nurses constantly reassess and reprioritize throughout their shifts. They remain alert to changes, gather new information, and adjust their plans accordingly. This continuous cycle of assessment, planning, intervention, and evaluation is at the heart of nursing practice.

The Dynamic Nature of Priorities

Consider this scenario: You arrive for your morning shift on a medical-surgical unit and receive report on four patients. Based on the information you receive, you create a mental plan for your first round of assessments. Patient A had an uneventful night and is scheduled for discharge. Patient B is post-operative day one and needs pain management. Patient C has newly elevated blood pressure readings. Patient D is a new admission arriving in 30 minutes.

You decide to assess Patient C first because of the blood pressure concern. But as you walk toward that room, you hear Patient B calling out in distress. Do you continue to Patient C or stop for Patient B?

The answer depends on what you observe and assess in that moment. Priorities shift based on real-time information. This is what makes prioritization dynamic—and why rigid, inflexible thinking can be dangerous in nursing.

1.3 Why Prioritization Matters

Patient Safety

The most compelling reason to master prioritization is patient safety. When nurses fail to recognize and respond to the most urgent patient needs, the consequences can be severe.

Failure to Rescue

Failure to rescue occurs when a patient deteriorates and the healthcare team does not recognize or respond to warning signs in time to prevent a serious adverse outcome, including death. Research has shown that many in-hospital cardiac arrests and deaths are preceded by warning signs that were either missed or not acted upon quickly enough (CITE: Aiken et al. or similar research on failure to rescue).

Prioritization is directly linked to rescue. A nurse who correctly identifies a patient at risk of deterioration and intervenes promptly can prevent a crisis. A nurse who is distracted by lower-priority tasks may miss critical cues until it is too late.

Missed Deterioration

Patients often do not deteriorate suddenly without warning. More commonly, there is a period of subtle changes—slightly increased heart rate, mild confusion, marginally decreased urine output—that precede a major event. Nurses who prioritize ongoing assessment and recognize patterns of deterioration can intervene early, when treatments are most effective.

Adverse Events

Adverse events include medication errors, falls, hospital-acquired infections, and other preventable harms. While not all adverse events are related to prioritization, many occur when nurses are overwhelmed, rushed, or focused on the wrong tasks. Effective prioritization helps nurses allocate their time and attention to the interventions most likely to prevent harm.

Nurse Well-Being

Prioritization is not only about patient outcomes—it also affects nurses themselves. Nurses who struggle to prioritize often feel overwhelmed, anxious, and out of control. They may stay late to finish documentation, skip breaks, or experience chronic stress that leads to burnout.

In contrast, nurses who develop strong prioritization skills report greater confidence and job satisfaction. They can manage their workload more effectively, leave on time more often, and experience less of the chaos that contributes to burnout. Prioritization is a form of self-care as much as it is a patient care skill.

Healthcare System Efficiency

When individual nurses prioritize effectively, the entire healthcare system benefits. Patients move through the system more smoothly. Lengths of stay decrease when complications are prevented. Resources are used more efficiently when the right care is delivered at the right time.

Legal and Ethical Obligations

Nurses have a professional and legal duty to provide competent care. This includes the ability to recognize urgent situations and respond appropriately. A nurse who fails to prioritize a deteriorating patient may face not only the emotional burden of a poor outcome but also professional discipline or legal liability.

The American Nurses Association Code of Ethics emphasizes the nurse's primary commitment to the patient. Meeting this commitment requires the ability to identify what each patient needs most and to act accordingly (CITE: ANA Code of Ethics).

1.4 Clinical Judgment and Prioritization

Prioritization does not happen in isolation. It is part of a larger process called clinical judgment—the ability to make sound decisions in complex, uncertain clinical situations.

The NCSBN Clinical Judgment Measurement Model

The National Council of State Boards of Nursing (NCSBN) developed the Clinical Judgment Measurement Model (NCJMM) to describe how nurses think through clinical situations. This model has become the foundation for the Next Generation NCLEX (NGN), which began testing candidates in 2023 (CITE: NCSBN, 2019 - Clinical Judgment Measurement Model).

The model includes six cognitive processes:

1. Recognize Cues

The first step is noticing relevant information. This includes data from assessment findings, vital signs, laboratory values, patient statements, and observations of behavior or appearance. Novice nurses often struggle to distinguish significant cues from background noise. With experience, nurses develop pattern recognition that allows them to quickly identify what matters.

2. Analyze Cues

Once cues are recognized, the nurse must interpret their meaning. What does it mean that this patient's blood pressure has dropped 20 points since the last reading? Is the patient's confusion new or baseline? Analyzing cues requires connecting observations to underlying knowledge of pathophysiology, pharmacology, and normal versus abnormal findings.

3. Prioritize Hypotheses

Based on the analysis, the nurse generates possible explanations for what is happening and ranks them by likelihood and urgency. If a post-surgical patient has new-onset confusion, possible hypotheses might include hypoxia, medication effect, infection, or blood glucose abnormality. Prioritizing these hypotheses helps focus the next steps.

4. Generate Solutions

The nurse identifies potential interventions to address the prioritized hypotheses. This might include actions the nurse can take independently, actions that require a provider order, or resources that need to be mobilized.

5. Take Action

The nurse implements the most appropriate interventions. In urgent situations, this may mean acting quickly while continuing to gather information. The ability to act decisively—while remaining open to new data—is a hallmark of expert nursing practice.

6. Evaluate Outcomes

After taking action, the nurse assesses the results. Did the intervention work? Is the patient improving, stable, or worsening? Evaluation leads back to recognizing new cues, and the cycle continues.

How the NCLEX Tests Clinical Judgment

The Next Generation NCLEX uses new item types designed to assess clinical judgment, including prioritization. You may encounter questions that ask you to:

- Highlight relevant assessment findings from a chart or nurse's notes
- Identify the most likely explanation for a set of symptoms
- Determine which patient should be seen first
- Sequence nursing actions in order of priority
- Evaluate whether an intervention was effective

Understanding the Clinical Judgment Measurement Model will help you approach these questions systematically rather than relying on guesswork.

1.5 The Novice-to-Expert Continuum

If prioritization feels difficult right now, that is completely normal. Research by Patricia Benner demonstrated that nurses progress through predictable stages as they develop clinical expertise (CITE: Benner, 1984 - From Novice to Expert).

Stages of Nursing Development

Novice

Novice nurses have little or no experience in the situations they encounter. They rely heavily on rules and guidelines because they lack the context to know when rules should be modified. Prioritization is particularly challenging because novices have not yet developed the pattern recognition that allows experienced nurses to quickly identify urgent situations.

Advanced Beginner

With some experience, nurses begin to recognize recurring patterns. They can identify meaningful aspects of situations but still have difficulty seeing the big picture. Prioritization improves, but advanced beginners may still struggle when situations do not fit familiar patterns.

Competent

Competent nurses, typically with two to three years of experience, can see their actions in terms of long-range goals. They can prioritize and manage multiple patients more effectively. However, they may still lack the speed and flexibility of more experienced nurses.

Proficient

Proficient nurses perceive situations as wholes rather than collections of parts. They recognize when a situation deviates from normal and can quickly zero in on the problem. Prioritization becomes more intuitive.

Expert

Expert nurses have an intuitive grasp of clinical situations. They no longer rely on rules or analytical processes in familiar situations—they simply know what to do. Their prioritization appears effortless because it is based on deep pattern recognition developed over years of practice.

Why Students Need Frameworks

As a nursing student or new graduate, you are likely in the novice or advanced beginner stage. You have not yet developed the pattern recognition that experts possess. This is not a character flaw—it is simply where you are in your development.

The good news is that you do not have to wait years to develop prioritization skills. Frameworks and systematic approaches can accelerate your learning. By applying structured methods like the ABCs, Maslow's Hierarchy of Needs, or the acute-versus-chronic comparison, you give yourself a reliable process to follow when your intuition has not yet developed.

Think of frameworks as training wheels. They provide stability while you are learning. As you gain experience, you will internalize these approaches and begin to prioritize more automatically. But even expert nurses fall back on explicit frameworks when they encounter unfamiliar or highly complex situations.

Building Confidence Through Practice

Prioritization skills improve with deliberate practice. Each time you work through a clinical scenario—whether in simulation, clinical rotation, or a workbook like this one—you strengthen your ability to recognize patterns and make sound decisions.

Do not be discouraged by mistakes. Every nurse, no matter how experienced, can recall situations where they wish they had prioritized differently. What matters is that you learn from each experience and continue to refine your approach.

1.6 Key Takeaways

- **Prioritization is dynamic and ongoing.** You will reassess and reprioritize constantly throughout every shift. Patient conditions change, new information emerges, and your plan must adapt accordingly.
- **Patient safety is always the primary concern.** When deciding what to do first, the question is always: What does my patient need most right now to stay safe?
- **Clinical judgment develops over time but can be accelerated with frameworks.** You are not expected to have expert intuition as a student. Use structured approaches to guide your decision-making while your pattern recognition develops.
- **The NCLEX tests prioritization through the lens of clinical judgment.** Understanding the Clinical Judgment Measurement Model will help you approach exam questions systematically and perform well on the Next Generation NCLEX.

1.7 Practice Problems

Directions: Select the best answer for each question. Answers and rationales are provided in the Answer Key.

1. Which statement best describes prioritization in nursing practice?

A. A one-time decision made at the beginning of each shift
B. A continuous process of reassessing and reordering patient needs
C. A skill that only experienced nurses can perform effectively
D. A task that should be delegated to the charge nurse

2. A nursing student asks the instructor why prioritization is considered a patient safety issue. Which response by the instructor is most accurate?

A. "Prioritization helps nurses finish their tasks before the end of the shift."
B. "Effective prioritization can prevent failure to rescue by ensuring early recognition of deterioration."
C. "Prioritization is mainly important for avoiding legal liability."
D. "Only critical care nurses need to worry about prioritization affecting safety."

3. According to the NCSBN Clinical Judgment Measurement Model, which cognitive process involves identifying relevant information from assessment data?

A. Analyze cues
B. Recognize cues
C. Prioritize hypotheses
D. Generate solutions

4. A nurse receives report on four patients at the start of the shift. Which approach to prioritization reflects best practice?

A. Complete all tasks for the first patient before moving to the second patient
B. Follow the same assessment order every day regardless of patient status
C. Assess the most unstable patient first, then reassess priorities based on findings
D. Ask the nursing assistant to assess all patients and report back

5. A new graduate nurse tells the preceptor, "I don't understand how you always know which patient to see first. It seems like instinct." Based on Benner's novice-to-expert theory, which response by the preceptor is most appropriate?

A. "You either have the instinct or you don't. It can't be taught."

B. "I've developed pattern recognition over years of experience. Frameworks can help you until you develop that same intuition."

C. "Just follow the ABCs for every situation and you'll be fine."

D. "Prioritization isn't really that important once you get faster at your tasks."

6. The nurse is caring for a patient whose blood pressure has decreased from 128/78 to 102/64 over the past two hours. The patient appears comfortable and is watching television. Using the Clinical Judgment Measurement Model, which step should the nurse take first?

A. Take action by calling the healthcare provider immediately

B. Generate solutions by preparing IV fluids

C. Analyze cues by considering possible reasons for the blood pressure change

D. Evaluate outcomes by checking if previous interventions were effective

7. A nurse on a busy medical-surgical unit has the following tasks to complete. Which reflects the highest priority?

A. Document the morning assessment findings

B. Respond to a patient's call light requesting pain medication

C. Check on a patient who was just reported to have new-onset confusion

D. Prepare discharge instructions for a patient leaving in two hours

8. Which factor best explains why nursing students often find prioritization challenging?

A. Nursing students are not intelligent enough to prioritize

B. Prioritization cannot be learned and must be innate

C. Nursing students lack the clinical experience needed for pattern recognition

D. Schools do not teach any prioritization content

9. A patient who was stable earlier in the shift now has oxygen saturation of 89% on room air and is using accessory muscles to breathe. The nurse had planned to complete medication administration for another patient. What should the nurse do?

A. Finish the medication administration since it was already planned

B. Ask the nursing assistant to check on the patient with low oxygen saturation

C. Immediately reprioritize and assess the patient with respiratory changes

D. Document the findings and notify the healthcare provider at the end of the shift

10. The nursing instructor is explaining the Next Generation NCLEX to students. Which statement about the exam is accurate?

A. "The NGN only tests memorization of facts and medication dosages."

B. "Clinical judgment questions ask you to recognize, analyze, and prioritize information."

C. "Prioritization questions have been removed from the current exam."

D. "The NGN does not require any critical thinking skills."

11. A nurse working in a long-term care facility receives word that a patient has fallen. At the same time, another patient's family member asks to discuss the plan of care. How should the nurse prioritize?

A. Speak with the family member first since they have been waiting

B. Ask another nurse to assess the fallen patient while continuing the family conversation

C. Immediately assess the patient who fell for injuries, then address the family's questions

D. Complete documentation of current tasks before responding to either situation

12. Which scenario demonstrates the dynamic nature of prioritization?

A. A nurse completes assessments on all patients in room number order every day

B. A nurse changes the plan to see a different patient first after learning of new chest pain

C. A nurse refuses to adjust the schedule despite a patient's changing condition

D. A nurse delegates all prioritization decisions to the charge nurse

13. A patient with a history of chronic obstructive pulmonary disease (COPD) has an oxygen saturation of 90% on 2 liters nasal cannula. The patient states, "This is my normal." Which action by the nurse demonstrates appropriate clinical judgment?

A. Immediately increase oxygen to 4 liters and call a rapid response

B. Recognize that this oxygen saturation may be acceptable for this patient and assess further

C. Assume the pulse oximeter is malfunctioning and ignore the reading

D. Discontinue oxygen therapy since the patient says this is normal

14. A nursing student is overwhelmed by a clinical assignment with three patients. The student does not know where to begin. Which advice from the instructor would be most helpful?

A. "Just do whatever feels right—trust your gut."

B. "Start with the patient closest to the nursing station."

C. "Use a systematic framework to identify which patient has the most urgent needs."

D. "Ask the nursing assistant to tell you what to do."

15. According to the chapter, why is prioritization considered an ethical obligation for nurses?

A. The hospital administration requires it for efficiency

B. Nurses have a professional commitment to meet each patient's most important needs

C. Prioritization is only an ethical issue in emergency departments

D. The nursing code of ethics does not address prioritization

16. The nurse is caring for a patient who had abdominal surgery yesterday. Assessment findings include: pain level 6/10, blood pressure 118/72, temperature 99.1°F (37.3°C), and bowel sounds absent. Using the "recognize cues" step of clinical judgment, which findings are most relevant to report?

A. The blood pressure, because it indicates hypertension

B. The absent bowel sounds and pain level, which are expected post-operative findings that require monitoring

C. The temperature, because any elevation is always an emergency

D. None of these findings require recognition—they are all normal

17. An experienced nurse appears to make prioritization decisions quickly and automatically. According to Benner's framework, this most likely indicates the nurse is functioning at which level?

A. Novice

B. Advanced beginner

C. Competent

D. Expert

18. A nurse must choose between two tasks: hanging a scheduled IV antibiotic that is due now, or assessing a patient who just returned from a procedure. Which question best helps the nurse prioritize?

A. "Which task will take less time?"

B. "Which task does the nursing assistant prefer I complete first?"

C. "Which situation poses a greater risk to patient safety if delayed?"

D. "Which patient's family is most likely to complain?"

19. The nurse is teaching a group of nursing students about prioritization. Which statement by a student indicates a need for further teaching?

A. "Priorities can change throughout the shift based on patient conditions."

B. "The ABCs can help me determine what to assess first in an emergency."

C. "Once I make a prioritization decision, I should stick with it no matter what."

D. "Clinical judgment involves analyzing cues and generating solutions."

20. A nurse receives report that includes the following information about a patient: "Blood pressure has been trending down overnight, urine output decreased, and the patient seems more tired than yesterday." Using clinical judgment, the nurse should:

A. Assume these are unrelated findings and assess the patient last

B. Recognize these as potentially significant cues that warrant prompt assessment

C. Wait for the healthcare provider to round before taking any action

D. Delegate the assessment to the nursing assistant

End of Chapter 1 Practice Problems

CHAPTER 2

Priority Frameworks

2.1 Learning Objectives

By the end of this chapter, you will be able to:

- Apply the ABCs framework to emergency and non-emergency situations
- Use Maslow's Hierarchy of Needs to establish patient priorities
- Differentiate between acute/chronic and actual/potential problems
- Select the appropriate framework based on clinical context

2.2 The ABCs: Airway, Breathing, Circulation

When a patient's life is in immediate danger, you need a framework that cuts through complexity and points you toward the most critical intervention. The ABCs—Airway, Breathing, Circulation—provide exactly that. This framework has been the gold standard in emergency care for decades, and for good reason: it addresses the physiological priorities that determine whether a patient lives or dies in the next few minutes.

The Logic Behind the ABCs

The ABCs follow a logical sequence based on how quickly each system failure leads to death:

Airway comes first because without a patent airway, oxygen cannot reach the lungs. Complete airway obstruction causes death within minutes. An unconscious patient whose tongue has fallen back, a choking victim, or a trauma patient with facial injuries and blood in the airway—all require immediate airway intervention before anything else matters.

Breathing is second because even with an open airway, the patient must be able to ventilate. A patient in severe respiratory distress, someone who has stopped breathing, or a patient with a tension pneumothorax needs breathing support immediately after the airway is secured.

Circulation is third because once oxygen is entering the lungs, it must be delivered to the tissues. Massive hemorrhage, cardiac arrest, or profound shock all threaten circulation. Without adequate perfusion, organs begin to fail within minutes.

Airway Priorities

When assessing airway, ask yourself: Is air able to move freely into and out of the lungs?

Signs of airway compromise include:

- Stridor (high-pitched sound indicating upper airway obstruction)
- Gurgling (fluid in the airway)
- Snoring respirations (tongue or soft tissue obstruction)
- Inability to speak or cry
- Choking or clutching at the throat
- Cyanosis (late sign)

Airway emergencies include:

- Complete or partial obstruction from a foreign body
- Anaphylaxis with throat swelling
- Trauma to the face, neck, or airway
- Decreased level of consciousness with loss of protective reflexes
- Aspiration risk in patients who cannot protect their airway

Breathing Priorities

Once the airway is patent, assess breathing: Is the patient ventilating adequately?

Signs of breathing problems include:

- Absent or diminished breath sounds
- Respiratory rate outside normal range (too fast or too slow)
- Use of accessory muscles
- Nasal flaring
- Paradoxical chest movement
- Oxygen saturation below acceptable range
- Cyanosis
- Altered mental status from hypoxia

Breathing emergencies include:

- Respiratory arrest
- Severe asthma or COPD exacerbation
- Pneumothorax (especially tension pneumothorax)
- Pulmonary embolism
- Acute pulmonary edema
- Opioid overdose with respiratory depression

Circulation Priorities

With airway and breathing addressed, assess circulation: Is oxygenated blood reaching the tissues?

Signs of circulatory compromise include:

- Absent or weak pulses
- Hypotension
- Tachycardia (early compensatory sign)
- Bradycardia (late or ominous sign)
- Pale, cool, clammy skin
- Delayed capillary refill
- Decreased urine output
- Altered mental status
- Active hemorrhage

Circulatory emergencies include:

- Cardiac arrest
- Hemorrhagic shock
- Cardiogenic shock
- Septic shock
- Severe dehydration
- Massive blood loss

Extended: ABCDE

Some clinical settings extend the framework to ABCDE:

D – Disability refers to neurological status. After addressing life-threatening ABC problems, assess the patient's level of consciousness, pupil response, and gross motor function. A quick assessment might use AVPU (Alert, responds to Voice, responds to Pain, Unresponsive) or the Glasgow Coma Scale.

E – Exposure means fully exposing the patient to identify all injuries or problems, particularly in trauma. This includes removing clothing to assess for wounds, rashes, or other findings that might be hidden—while also preventing hypothermia.

When to Use the ABCs

The ABCs are your go-to framework in these situations:

- **Cardiac or respiratory arrest**: The ABCs guide your BLS and ACLS response
- **Rapid Response or Code Blue**: Systematic assessment of immediately life-threatening problems

- **Trauma**: Primary survey uses ABCDE to identify and treat the most lethal injuries first
- **Emergency department triage**: Identifying patients who need immediate intervention
- **Any acute deterioration**: When a patient suddenly worsens, start with ABCs
- **Multiple patients in crisis**: ABCs help you determine who needs you first

When ABCs May Not Apply

The ABCs are designed for emergencies. In non-emergent situations, other frameworks may be more appropriate. For example:

- A stable patient with multiple chronic conditions might be better prioritized using Maslow's hierarchy
- A patient whose physical needs are met but who is anxious about surgery needs psychosocial support, not ABC assessment
- Routine morning assessments on stable patients do not require emergency-style prioritization

The key is recognizing when you are in an emergency versus a non-emergent situation, and selecting the appropriate framework.

2.3 Maslow's Hierarchy of Needs

While the ABCs excel in emergencies, many clinical situations involve patients whose lives are not in immediate danger but who have multiple competing needs. Abraham Maslow's Hierarchy of Needs, originally published in 1943, provides a framework for understanding human motivation that nurses have adapted for prioritizing patient care (Maslow, 1943).

The Five Levels

Maslow proposed that human needs exist in a hierarchy, with more basic needs requiring satisfaction before higher-level needs become important:

Level 1: Physiological Needs

These are the most basic survival needs: oxygen, water, food, elimination, sleep, temperature regulation, and freedom from pain. In nursing terms, this level includes airway, breathing, circulation, nutrition, hydration, elimination, and comfort. These needs take priority because without them, the body cannot survive.

Level 2: Safety and Security

Once physiological needs are met, people seek safety—both physical safety from harm and psychological security from fear and anxiety. In healthcare, this includes fall prevention, infection control, medication safety, protection from abuse, and helping patients feel secure in an unfamiliar environment.

Level 3: Love and Belonging

Humans are social beings who need connection with others. Patients need contact with family and friends, spiritual support, and a sense of being cared for. Isolation and loneliness can impair healing and well-being.

Level 4: Esteem

People need to feel valued, competent, and respected. For patients, this includes maintaining dignity, being involved in care decisions, achieving health goals, and preserving independence when possible.

Level 5: Self-Actualization

The highest level involves reaching one's full potential—growth, creativity, and meaning. For patients, this might involve adjusting to a new health reality, finding purpose despite illness, or achieving personal goals.

Applying Maslow to Nursing Prioritization

The principle is straightforward: **address lower-level needs before higher-level needs**. A patient cannot focus on learning about diabetes management (esteem/self-actualization) if they are in pain (physiological) or afraid they will fall (safety).

Example 1: A patient is one day post-hip replacement. She has pain rated 7/10, needs to ambulate for the first time, and her daughter wants to discuss discharge plans.

Using Maslow:

- Pain (physiological) comes first—medicate for pain
- Safe ambulation (safety) comes second—assist with physical therapy once pain is controlled
- Discharge planning discussion (potentially involving esteem and self-actualization) comes third

Example 2: A nurse has three patients to assess at the start of shift:

- Patient A: Stable vital signs, requesting information about a new diagnosis
- Patient B: Complaining of chest pain rated 4/10
- Patient C: Anxious about upcoming surgery, wants to talk

Using Maslow:

- Patient B has a physiological need (chest pain) that must be assessed first
- Patient C has safety/security needs (anxiety) that come second
- Patient A has learning needs (esteem/self-actualization) that can wait until the others are addressed

Limitations of Maslow's Hierarchy

While Maslow's framework is useful, it has limitations:

Not always linear: Real patients do not always progress neatly through the hierarchy. A dying patient may prioritize saying goodbye to family (love/belonging) over aggressive treatment of physiological symptoms. A patient with chronic pain may have adapted and prioritize other needs.

Cultural variations: Different cultures may prioritize needs differently. Some patients may place family or spiritual needs above personal comfort. Respect patient values even when they do not align perfectly with the hierarchy.

Concurrent needs: Patients often have needs at multiple levels simultaneously. A patient may be in pain (physiological), afraid of falling (safety), and lonely (belonging) all at once. The hierarchy helps you sequence your interventions, but you must address all relevant needs.

Not designed for emergencies: Maslow's hierarchy is better suited for ongoing care of stable patients than for acute crises. In an emergency, use the ABCs.

2.4 Acute vs. Chronic Conditions

Another essential framework for prioritization compares acute and chronic conditions. The principle is simple: **acute problems generally take priority over chronic problems**.

Defining Acute and Chronic

Acute conditions are new onset, rapidly developing, or unstable. They represent a change from the patient's baseline and often require immediate intervention. Acute conditions are time-sensitive—delays in treatment can lead to deterioration.

Chronic conditions are long-standing, slowly progressive, and typically stable. The patient has been living with the condition, and while it requires ongoing management, it is not an immediate threat.

The Change from Baseline Principle

One of the most important concepts in nursing assessment is recognizing **change from baseline**. A finding that would be alarming in one patient might be normal for another:

- Blood pressure of 88/60 is concerning in most patients but might be normal for a young athlete
- Oxygen saturation of 89% is alarming for most patients but might be baseline for someone with severe COPD
- Confusion in a previously alert patient is urgent; chronic confusion in a patient with dementia is baseline

When you notice a change from baseline, it signals an acute problem requiring priority attention. When a finding is consistent with the patient's usual status, it may represent a chronic condition that, while important, does not demand immediate action.

Examples of Acute vs. Chronic Prioritization

Example 1: A patient has both chronic back pain (ongoing for years) and new-onset chest pain (started 30 minutes ago).

- The chest pain is acute and takes priority
- The chronic back pain, while real and important, can be addressed after the acute problem is evaluated

Example 2: A patient with a history of well-controlled hypertension now has a blood pressure of 198/110 with headache and blurred vision.

- This represents acute severe hypertension (hypertensive urgency or emergency)—a change from the patient's usual controlled state

- It takes priority over routine management of the chronic condition

Example 3: A nurse is caring for two patients:

- Patient A: Long-standing diabetes with blood glucose currently 186 mg/dL (typical for this patient)
- Patient B: New-onset confusion in a patient who was oriented earlier today
- Patient B's acute change in mental status takes priority over Patient A's chronic, stable glucose elevation

Unstable vs. Stable

Related to acute vs. chronic is the concept of **unstable vs. stable**:

- **Unstable** patients have vital signs or conditions that are fluctuating, worsening, or not responding to treatment. They require close monitoring and may deteriorate.
- **Stable** patients have consistent vital signs and conditions that are responding appropriately to treatment. They are at lower risk for immediate deterioration.

Unstable patients take priority over stable patients, regardless of diagnosis. A patient with a "minor" condition who is unstable needs attention before a patient with a "serious" diagnosis who is currently stable.

2.5 Actual vs. Potential Problems

Nursing diagnosis frameworks distinguish between actual problems (currently occurring) and potential problems (risk for). This distinction helps with prioritization.

Actual Problems

Actual problems are present right now. The patient is experiencing the condition, and assessment data confirms its existence.

Examples:

- Acute pain (the patient reports pain, displays pain behaviors)
- Impaired skin integrity (there is a visible wound)
- Ineffective airway clearance (the patient cannot clear secretions)
- Fluid volume deficit (signs of dehydration are present)

Actual problems require intervention to resolve or manage what is already happening.

Potential Problems (Risk For)

Potential problems are not yet present but could develop based on risk factors. The patient has characteristics that increase their likelihood of developing the problem.

Examples:

- Risk for falls (patient has unsteady gait, takes sedating medications)

- Risk for infection (patient has an IV line, surgical incision)
- Risk for impaired skin integrity (patient is immobile, incontinent)
- Risk for aspiration (patient has dysphagia, decreased consciousness)

Potential problems require preventive interventions to stop the problem from occurring.

Prioritization Principle

The general rule: **Actual problems take priority over potential problems.**

If a patient has acute pain (actual) and risk for falls (potential), address the pain first. The pain is happening now; the fall has not occurred yet.

However, there are important exceptions:

Exception 1: Imminent risk with severe consequences

If a potential problem is highly likely to occur imminently and would cause serious harm, prevention may take priority. For example, if a confused patient is climbing out of bed and about to fall, fall prevention is the immediate priority—even though no fall has occurred yet.

Exception 2: Quick preventive action

Sometimes preventing a potential problem takes only seconds. Raising side rails to reduce fall risk while passing by the room does not delay care for actual problems.

Exception 3: Actual problem is low severity

If the actual problem is minor and the potential problem is severe, you might prioritize prevention. A patient with mild, chronic constipation (actual) who is at high risk for aspiration during feeding (potential) should have aspiration precautions implemented first.

Practical Application

When you have multiple patients or multiple problems, ask yourself:

1. What is actually happening right now? (Actual problems)

2. What could happen if I do not intervene? (Potential problems)

3. Which actual problems are most urgent?

4. Which potential problems are most imminent or have the worst consequences?

This systematic approach helps you sequence your care appropriately.

2.6 Choosing the Right Framework

With multiple frameworks available, how do you know which one to use? The answer depends on the clinical situation.

Decision Guide

Is this a life-threatening emergency?

→ Use **ABCs**

When a patient is in cardiac arrest, respiratory failure, choking, or showing signs of shock, do not deliberate—go straight to ABCs. This framework is designed for situations where death is imminent without immediate intervention.

Am I prioritizing across multiple patients with various non-emergent needs?

→ Use **Maslow's Hierarchy**

When you have several stable patients and need to decide who to see first or which needs to address first, Maslow's provides a systematic way to rank needs from basic survival to higher-order needs.

Am I comparing two or more problems in the same patient?

→ Use **Acute vs. Chronic** or **Actual vs. Potential**

When a single patient has multiple issues and you need to decide which to address first, these frameworks help you sort immediate, pressing problems from longer-standing or not-yet-manifested ones.

Am I unsure of the situation?

→ Start with **ABCs** to rule out life threats, then apply other frameworks

When in doubt, a quick ABC assessment ensures you have not missed an emergency. Once you confirm the patient is not in immediate danger, you can use Maslow or other frameworks for further prioritization.

Combining Frameworks

In reality, you will often combine frameworks. Consider this scenario:

You are a nurse on a medical-surgical unit with four patients. You receive word that:

- Patient A has oxygen saturation of 84% (down from 95% an hour ago)
- Patient B is requesting pain medication
- Patient C wants to discuss discharge concerns
- Patient D, who is at risk for falls, is trying to get out of bed unassisted

How do you prioritize?

Step 1: ABCs — Patient A has a breathing problem (oxygen saturation 84%). This is the top priority because it is potentially life-threatening.

Step 2: Actual vs. Potential — Patient D is about to fall (imminent risk with serious consequences). Even though no fall has occurred, prevention is urgent. This is your second priority.

Step 3: Maslow — Between Patient B (pain, a physiological need) and Patient C (discharge concerns, a higher-level need), Patient B takes priority.

Final sequence: A → D → B → C

This example shows how frameworks work together. You did not choose just one; you applied the most relevant framework to each component of the decision.

Flexibility and Clinical Judgment

Frameworks are tools, not rigid rules. They guide your thinking but do not replace clinical judgment. There will be situations where the "correct" answer according to a framework does not feel right—and you may be picking up on something important.

For example, a framework might suggest that a patient with mild pain takes priority over a patient who "just seems off." But experienced nurses know that the patient who "seems off" may be showing early signs of serious deterioration. Trust your instincts, but use frameworks to check your reasoning and ensure you have not missed something obvious.

2.7 Framework Comparison Table

Framework	Best Used When	Key Principle	Example
ABCs (Airway, Breathing, Circulation)	Emergency situations; immediate threat to life	Address life-threatening problems in ABC order	Cardiac arrest, respiratory failure, hemorrhagic shock
Maslow's Hierarchy of Needs	Multiple patients or needs; non-emergent prioritization	Lower-level needs (physiological, safety) before higher-level needs	Prioritizing morning assessments across a patient assignment
Acute vs. Chronic	Comparing conditions in one patient or across patients	Acute, new-onset, or unstable problems before chronic, stable problems	New chest pain takes priority over chronic back pain
Actual vs. Potential	Determining priority among nursing diagnoses or interventions	Actual (occurring now) before potential (risk for)—with exceptions for imminent, severe risk	Current pain before fall risk—unless patient is actively about to fall

2.8 Practice Problems

Directions: Select the best answer for each question. Answers and rationales are provided in the Answer Key.

1. A nurse responds to a patient who has fallen and is lying on the floor, unresponsive. Using the ABCs framework, what should the nurse assess first?

A. Check for bleeding from injuries sustained in the fall

B. Determine if the patient's airway is patent

C. Assess circulation by checking for a pulse

D. Call for help before performing any assessment

2. According to Maslow's Hierarchy of Needs, which patient need should take priority?

A. A patient who wants to learn about managing a new diagnosis

B. A patient who is experiencing moderate incisional pain

C. A patient who feels isolated and wants family to visit

D. A patient who is anxious about loss of independence

3. A nurse is caring for a patient with a history of chronic obstructive pulmonary disease (COPD) who normally has an oxygen saturation of 89-91% on 2L nasal cannula. Today, the patient's oxygen saturation is 88% on the same oxygen setting. How should the nurse interpret this finding?

A. This is an emergency requiring immediate intervention with the ABCs

B. This is a significant change from baseline requiring prompt assessment

C. This is within the patient's normal range and does not require action

D. This indicates the patient's COPD is worsening and requires hospice referral

4. A patient on a medical unit has the following needs: constipation for the past two days, new-onset shortness of breath, and a request to speak with the chaplain. Using prioritization frameworks, in what order should the nurse address these needs?

A. Constipation, shortness of breath, chaplain visit

B. Chaplain visit, shortness of breath, constipation

C. Shortness of breath, constipation, chaplain visit

D. Shortness of breath, chaplain visit, constipation

5. A patient with heart failure is admitted with acute shortness of breath. Which assessment finding would the nurse address as the highest priority?

A. Bilateral lower extremity edema

B. Weight gain of 5 pounds over the past week

C. Oxygen saturation of 82% on room air

D. Elevated B-type natriuretic peptide (BNP) level

6. According to Maslow's Hierarchy, which level of needs must be addressed before a patient can focus on learning self-care for a new colostomy?

A. Self-actualization needs

B. Esteem needs

C. Physiological and safety needs

D. Love and belonging needs

7. A nurse is prioritizing care for four patients. Which patient should be assessed first?

A. A patient with chronic kidney disease who has a potassium level of 5.2 mEq/L (stable for this patient)

B. A patient with pneumonia who has new-onset confusion and temperature of 102.8°F (39.3°C)

C. A patient with diabetes who has a blood glucose of 198 mg/dL before breakfast

D. A patient who is post-operative day 2 and reports incisional pain of 4/10

8. A nurse is caring for a patient who has both acute pain (rated 8/10) and a risk for infection due to an IV site. Using the actual vs. potential problem framework, which should the nurse address first?

A. The risk for infection, because prevention is more important than treatment

B. The acute pain, because actual problems take priority over potential problems

C. Both should be addressed simultaneously by two different nurses

D. Neither is a priority because the patient is stable

9. Which scenario best demonstrates appropriate use of the ABCs framework?

A. A nurse uses ABCs to decide which stable patient to assess first during morning rounds

B. A nurse uses ABCs to guide assessment of a patient found unresponsive in bed

C. A nurse uses ABCs to determine whether a patient needs pain medication before ambulation

D. A nurse uses ABCs to prioritize patient education about medication side effects

10. A patient with a history of falls is trying to climb out of bed without assistance. At the same time, the nurse receives a call that another patient is requesting a scheduled pain medication. What should the nurse do first?

A. Administer the pain medication because it is a scheduled treatment

B. Ensure the patient at risk for falls is safe, then address the pain medication request

C. Ask the unlicensed assistive personnel to give the pain medication

D. Document both requests and address them at the end of the medication pass

11. Which statement best describes the "change from baseline" principle in prioritization?

A. All patients should be assessed using the same normal values regardless of history

B. Findings that represent a change from a patient's usual status may indicate an acute problem

C. Chronic conditions should always be addressed before acute conditions

D. Baseline values should be ignored in emergency situations

12. A nurse is teaching a nursing student about Maslow's Hierarchy of Needs. Which statement by the student indicates understanding?

A. "A patient in severe pain will be able to focus on learning about their medications."

B. "Safety needs are more basic than physiological needs."

C. "I should address a patient's physiological needs before focusing on their emotional needs."

D. "Self-actualization is the most basic human need."

13. A patient is admitted with acute appendicitis and is scheduled for surgery. The patient also has well-controlled type 2 diabetes and chronic lower back pain. Which problem should be the nurse's highest priority?

A. The chronic lower back pain because it affects quality of life

B. The type 2 diabetes because it can cause surgical complications

C. The acute appendicitis because it is an acute, potentially life-threatening condition

D. All three problems should be addressed with equal priority

14. During morning rounds, a nurse assesses four patients. Which patient has the highest priority based on the ABCs framework?

A. A patient who is anxious about a procedure scheduled for later today

B. A patient with crackles in bilateral lung bases and oxygen saturation of 91%

C. A patient reporting nausea after taking morning medications

D. A patient with a blood pressure of 142/88 mmHg

15. A nurse is caring for a patient who is refusing to eat because they are depressed about a new cancer diagnosis. According to Maslow's Hierarchy, how should the nurse approach this situation?

A. Focus only on the physiological need for nutrition and insist the patient eat

B. Recognize that emotional needs may be affecting physiological needs and address both

C. Ignore the nutritional concern until the patient's depression is resolved

D. Consult psychiatry before addressing any physical needs

16. Which patient situation represents a potential problem rather than an actual problem?

A. A patient with a stage 2 pressure injury on the sacrum

B. A patient who is immobile and has fragile skin

C. A patient with purulent drainage from a surgical incision

D. A patient with a blood glucose level of 52 mg/dL

17. A nurse is using the acute vs. chronic framework to prioritize care. Which patient should be seen first?

A. A patient with chronic heart failure who has 2+ pitting edema in the ankles (baseline for this patient)

B. A patient with chronic back pain who reports their usual pain level of 5/10

C. A patient with a history of anxiety who is having a panic attack with hyperventilation

D. A patient with well-controlled hypertension and current blood pressure of 138/86 mmHg

18. According to the chapter, when might a potential problem take priority over an actual problem?

A. When the potential problem is more interesting to the nurse

B. When the actual problem is minor and the potential problem is imminent with severe consequences

C. Potential problems should never take priority over actual problems

D. When the patient requests that the potential problem be addressed first

19. A nurse in the emergency department is triaging four patients who arrive simultaneously. Using prioritization frameworks, which patient should be seen first?

A. A 45-year-old with severe abdominal pain rated 9/10

B. A 30-year-old with a laceration to the forearm that is bleeding through the bandage

C. A 60-year-old who is unresponsive and not breathing

D. A 25-year-old with a possible fractured ankle after a fall

20. A nursing student asks why frameworks are helpful for prioritization. What is the best response?

A. "Frameworks replace the need for clinical judgment."

B. "Frameworks provide a systematic approach when you cannot rely on intuition alone."

C. "Frameworks should only be used by novice nurses; experts do not need them."

D. "Frameworks guarantee you will always make the correct prioritization decision."

End of Chapter 2 Practice Problems

CHAPTER 3

Principles of Delegation

3.1 Learning Objectives

By the end of this chapter, you will be able to:

- Define delegation and differentiate it from assignment
- Identify the Five Rights of Delegation
- Explain the legal and professional accountability in delegation
- Recognize barriers to effective delegation

3.2 Defining Delegation

Delegation is one of the most important—and most misunderstood—skills in nursing practice. As healthcare becomes increasingly complex and nurses manage larger patient loads, the ability to delegate effectively has become essential for safe, efficient care delivery. Yet many nurses, especially new graduates, struggle with delegation. They may feel guilty asking others to help, uncertain about what can be delegated, or worried about losing control over patient care.

Understanding what delegation actually means—and what it does not mean—is the first step toward becoming skilled at this essential nursing competency.

What Is Delegation?

The National Council of State Boards of Nursing (NCSBN) and the American Nurses Association (ANA) jointly define delegation as:

"The process for a nurse to direct another person to perform nursing tasks and activities."

More specifically, delegation involves transferring responsibility for performing a specific task to another person while retaining accountability for the outcome. The registered nurse authorizes a competent individual to perform a selected task in a selected situation under the nurse's supervision (NCSBN & ANA, 2019).

Several key elements are embedded in this definition:

Transfer of responsibility. When you delegate, you are asking someone else to take responsibility for completing a task. The delegatee accepts that responsibility when they agree to perform the task.

Retention of accountability. Even though you have transferred responsibility for the task, you remain accountable for the overall outcome. You cannot delegate accountability—it stays with you, the registered nurse.

Competent individual. Delegation requires that the person receiving the delegated task is competent to perform it. This means they have the knowledge, skills, and abilities needed, and that the task falls within their scope of practice or job description.

Supervision. Delegation occurs under the nurse's supervision. The type and intensity of supervision varies based on the task, the patient, and the delegatee's experience.

Delegation vs. Assignment

Many nurses use the terms "delegation" and "assignment" interchangeably, but they have distinct meanings:

Delegation involves transferring responsibility for a task to someone for whom the task is not part of their typical job duties—or transferring authority to perform nursing tasks that require the delegator's professional judgment to determine appropriateness.

Assignment refers to distributing work among team members where the work is already within each person's scope of practice and job description. Assignment involves routine distribution of expected duties.

Example of Assignment:

The charge nurse assigns the LPN to care for three stable patients on the unit. Providing care for stable patients is within the LPN's scope of practice and job description. This is assignment—distributing work that the LPN is already expected and authorized to perform.

Example of Delegation:

The RN asks the unlicensed assistive personnel (UAP) to obtain vital signs on a patient who has been showing signs of instability. Normally, the UAP obtains vital signs on stable patients as part of routine care. However, the RN is specifically delegating this task with particular instructions about what to watch for and when to report back immediately. The RN is transferring responsibility for this specific task while retaining accountability for recognizing whether the findings indicate a problem.

Why the Distinction Matters

Understanding the difference between delegation and assignment matters because it affects your legal and professional responsibilities:

- When you make an **assignment**, you are distributing work within established parameters. The person receiving the assignment is independently responsible for performing their job duties correctly.
- When you **delegate**, you are making a judgment that a specific task is appropriate for a specific person in a specific situation. You bear greater responsibility for ensuring the task is appropriate and for supervising its completion.

Both assignment and delegation require you to know the scope of practice and competencies of your team members. But delegation demands more active decision-making and closer supervision.

3.3 The Five Rights of Delegation

The NCSBN and ANA have established the Five Rights of Delegation as a framework to guide nurses in making safe delegation decisions (NCSBN & ANA, 2019). Just as the "Five Rights" of medication administration help prevent errors, the Five Rights of Delegation help ensure that tasks are delegated safely and appropriately.

Before delegating any task, the nurse should consider each of these five elements:

Right Task

Is this task appropriate to delegate?

Not all nursing tasks can be delegated. The right task is one that:

- Is within the delegatee's scope of practice or job description
- Does not require nursing judgment during its performance
- Is routine and predictable in nature
- Has a predictable outcome
- Does not require repeated nursing assessment throughout the task

Tasks that should NOT be delegated include:

- Initial patient assessment
- Nursing diagnosis and care planning
- Evaluation of patient progress
- Tasks requiring professional nursing judgment
- Patient education (initial teaching)
- Telephone orders from providers
- Triage decisions
- Any task the delegatee is not trained to perform

Tasks commonly appropriate for delegation to UAPs include:

- Vital signs on stable patients
- Activities of daily living (bathing, dressing, grooming)
- Ambulation of stable patients
- Intake and output measurement
- Routine specimen collection
- Feeding assistance
- Bed making and positioning
- Transport of stable patients

When considering whether a task is right for delegation, ask yourself: "Can this task be performed without ongoing nursing judgment?" If the answer is no, do not delegate it.

Right Circumstance

Is this the right situation for delegation?

Even tasks that can generally be delegated may not be appropriate in every circumstance. Consider:

Patient factors:

- Is the patient stable enough for this task to be delegated?
- Is the patient's condition predictable?
- Are there complicating factors that require nursing assessment during the task?
- Has the patient's condition changed recently?

Environmental factors:

- Is the setting appropriate for delegation?
- Are necessary resources and equipment available?
- Is adequate supervision available?
- Is this an emergency situation requiring RN presence?

Example: Obtaining vital signs is generally appropriate for delegation to a UAP. However, if the patient is showing early signs of sepsis and you need to closely monitor the response to treatment, you might choose to obtain the vital signs yourself—or provide very specific instructions about what to report and follow up quickly.

Right Person

Is this the right person to perform this task?

The right person has:

Appropriate licensure or certification. The task must fall within what this person is legally permitted to do. An LPN can perform many tasks that a UAP cannot. State law and facility policy define these boundaries.

Demonstrated competence. The person must have the knowledge and skills to perform the task correctly. This goes beyond licensure—have they actually been trained on this specific task? Have they demonstrated competence?

Availability and workload. Is this person available to perform the task in a timely manner? Do they have capacity, or are they already overwhelmed with other responsibilities?

Familiarity with the patient. While not always required, familiarity with the patient can enhance safety and efficiency.

Before delegating, ask yourself:

- "Is this person qualified to do this task?"
- "Has this person demonstrated that they can do this task correctly?"
- "Does state law and facility policy permit this person to do this task?"

If you are unsure about a team member's competency, do not delegate until you have verified their training and skills.

Right Directions and Communication

Have I communicated clearly and completely?

Delegation fails most often due to poor communication. The delegating nurse must provide clear, specific, and complete instructions. Effective delegation communication includes:

What task to perform. Be specific about exactly what you are asking the person to do.

For which patient. Clearly identify the patient by name and room number.

Timeline. When should the task be completed? Is it urgent, or can it be done within a certain timeframe?

Expected outcomes. What should the result be? What is normal for this patient?

What to report. Specify findings that should be reported immediately. Do not assume the delegatee knows what is significant.

When to report back. When do you expect to hear that the task is complete?

Opportunity for questions. Allow time for the delegatee to ask clarifying questions. Encourage them to speak up if something is unclear.

Example of clear delegation communication:

"Maria, I need you to get vital signs on Mr. Johnson in room 412. He's the patient recovering from hip surgery. Please get a full set—blood pressure, pulse, respirations, temperature, and oxygen saturation. He's been stable, but let me know right away if his blood pressure is below 100 systolic or his heart rate is over 100. I need these within the next 30 minutes. Do you have any questions?"

Example of poor delegation communication:

"Can you check on the guy in 412?"

The second example leaves too much to interpretation. What exactly should be checked? What findings are concerning? When is it needed?

Right Supervision and Evaluation

Am I providing appropriate oversight and follow-up?

Delegation does not end when you give instructions. You must provide appropriate supervision and evaluate the outcome.

Levels of supervision:

- **Direct supervision:** You are physically present and observe the task being performed. Used for new employees, unfamiliar tasks, or high-risk situations.
- **Indirect supervision:** You are available for questions and guidance but not directly observing. You monitor progress and evaluate outcomes. This is the most common supervision level for experienced staff.

Follow-up responsibilities:

- Check in at appropriate intervals based on the task and the patient's condition
- Verify that the task was completed
- Evaluate the outcome—was it done correctly? What was the patient's response?
- Provide feedback to the delegatee—both positive and constructive

More frequent follow-up is needed when:

- The delegatee is new or inexperienced
- The patient is unstable or unpredictable
- The task is complex or unfamiliar
- Problems have occurred with similar tasks in the past

Remember: You cannot evaluate what you do not monitor. Delegation without supervision is abandonment of your professional responsibility.

3.4 Accountability in Delegation

One of the most critical concepts in delegation is understanding who is accountable when things go wrong—or right. The principle is straightforward but often misunderstood:

The RN Is Always Accountable

The registered nurse is accountable for the decision to delegate. This includes:

- Assessing whether the task is appropriate for delegation
- Determining whether the patient's condition allows for delegation
- Selecting the right person to perform the task
- Providing adequate direction and communication
- Supervising appropriately
- Evaluating the outcome

If a delegation decision results in patient harm, the RN may be held accountable for making an inappropriate delegation decision—even if the actual error was made by the delegatee.

The Delegatee Is Responsible

The person performing the delegated task is responsible for their own actions. This includes:

- Accepting only tasks they are competent to perform
- Asking for clarification when instructions are unclear
- Performing the task correctly
- Reporting relevant findings to the RN
- Recognizing their own limitations and communicating them

If a UAP accepts a delegated task and performs it negligently, the UAP is responsible for their negligent actions. However, this does not eliminate the RN's accountability for the delegation decision itself.

You Cannot Delegate Accountability

A common phrase captures this principle: **"Delegate the task, not the responsibility."**

When you delegate, you transfer:

- Responsibility for performing the task
- Authority to complete the task

When you delegate, you retain:

- Accountability for the overall outcome
- Accountability for the delegation decision
- Responsibility for supervision and follow-up

This is why delegation requires careful judgment. You are placing your professional accountability on the line when you delegate. Choose wisely.

Shared Responsibility Model

In practice, delegation creates a chain of responsibility:

1. **The RN** is accountable for assessing, delegating, supervising, and evaluating

2. **The delegatee** is responsible for performing the task competently and reporting appropriately

3. **The organization** is responsible for ensuring adequate staffing, training, and policies

When errors occur, all three levels may share responsibility to varying degrees, depending on the circumstances.

3.5 Legal Considerations

Delegation is not just a matter of best practice—it has significant legal implications. Understanding the legal framework helps protect your patients, your license, and yourself.

State Nurse Practice Acts

State Nurse Practice Acts are the primary legal authority governing nursing practice, including delegation. Each state's Board of Nursing establishes rules about:

- What tasks can be delegated
- Who can receive delegated tasks
- What supervision is required
- What documentation is necessary

Key point: Delegation laws vary significantly by state. What is permitted in one state may be prohibited in another. As a nurse, you are responsible for knowing the delegation rules in your state.

For example:

- Some states allow UAPs to perform blood glucose monitoring; others do not
- Some states permit LPNs to administer IV push medications; others prohibit it
- Requirements for supervision of LPNs vary by state

When you move to a new state or work in a state different from where you were trained, verify the delegation rules before assuming practices from your previous location are acceptable.

Facility Policies

Facility policies may be more restrictive than state law. An employer can establish policies that limit delegation beyond what state law permits, but cannot expand delegation beyond legal limits.

For example, state law might permit UAPs to perform a certain task, but your hospital's policy might prohibit it due to risk management concerns. You must follow the more restrictive standard—in this case, the facility policy.

Always know your facility's delegation policies. If you are unsure, ask your supervisor or consult the policy manual before delegating.

Documentation Requirements

Proper documentation protects everyone involved in delegation. Depending on your facility's requirements, documentation may include:

- Tasks delegated and to whom
- Instructions provided
- Supervision and follow-up performed
- Outcomes and any complications
- Communication with the delegatee

Documentation provides evidence that delegation was appropriate and that proper supervision occurred. In a legal dispute, what is not documented may be assumed not to have happened.

Liability Considerations

When delegation leads to patient harm, liability may fall on multiple parties:

The RN may be liable for:

- Delegating a task that should not have been delegated
- Delegating to someone who was not competent
- Failing to provide adequate instructions
- Failing to supervise appropriately
- Failing to intervene when problems arose

The delegatee may be liable for:

- Accepting a task they were not competent to perform
- Failing to perform the task correctly
- Failing to report important findings
- Acting outside their scope of practice

The employer may be liable for:

- Inadequate staffing that forced inappropriate delegation
- Failure to train staff properly
- Failure to establish clear delegation policies
- Failure to enforce existing policies

Protecting yourself legally requires knowing the rules, following them carefully, documenting appropriately, and exercising sound professional judgment.

3.6 Barriers to Effective Delegation

Despite its importance, many nurses struggle to delegate effectively. Understanding common barriers can help you overcome them.

"I Can Do It Faster Myself"

This is perhaps the most common barrier. It may even be true—in the short term. However, consider:

- If you never delegate, you will always be overwhelmed
- Delegation develops team members' skills and confidence
- Time invested in teaching and delegating pays off in future efficiency
- Some tasks do not require your level of expertise

Fear of Burdening Others

Many nurses feel guilty asking colleagues to help. They worry about:

- Being seen as lazy or incompetent
- Adding to others' workloads
- Creating conflict or resentment

Remember: Delegation is not about avoiding work. It is about ensuring that the right person performs each task. Team members expect to receive delegated tasks—it is part of their role.

Lack of Trust in Team Members

Some nurses hesitate to delegate because they do not trust others to do the job correctly. This might stem from:

- Past experiences with errors
- Not knowing team members' competencies
- Perfectionism or need for control
- Genuine concerns about a specific individual's skills

If you have concerns about a team member's competence, address those concerns directly rather than refusing to delegate altogether. Verify training, provide education if needed, or escalate concerns to management.

Poor Communication Habits

Delegation requires clear communication, which takes effort. Barriers include:

- Rushing through instructions
- Assuming others know what you mean
- Not allowing time for questions
- Not following up

Improving communication skills improves delegation effectiveness.

Unclear Role Boundaries

When team members are unsure about their roles and responsibilities, delegation becomes difficult. Contributing factors include:

- Vague job descriptions
- Inconsistent expectations among nurses
- Lack of orientation for new staff
- Poor organizational communication

If role boundaries are unclear on your unit, work with your leadership to clarify expectations.

Inadequate Training

Delegation requires knowledge and skill. Many nurses receive little formal training in delegation during nursing school. If you feel unprepared to delegate, seek out:

- Continuing education on delegation
- Mentorship from experienced nurses
- Unit-specific guidance on delegation practices

Overcoming Barriers

Effective delegation is a skill that improves with practice. To develop your delegation skills:

1. Start with simple, low-risk tasks

2. Use the Five Rights framework consistently

3. Practice clear, complete communication

4. Follow up and provide feedback

5. Learn from mistakes without giving up

6. Gradually expand the complexity of delegated tasks

Remember that failing to delegate when appropriate is just as problematic as delegating inappropriately. Both can compromise patient care and overwhelm nursing staff.

3.7 Key Takeaways

- **Delegation is transferring responsibility for a task while retaining accountability for the outcome.** The RN authorizes a competent person to perform a specific task and supervises its completion.
- **Delegation differs from assignment.** Assignment involves distributing routine work within established scopes of practice; delegation involves transferring authority for tasks that require nursing judgment to determine appropriateness.
- **The Five Rights of Delegation guide safe delegation decisions:** Right Task, Right Circumstance, Right Person, Right Directions and Communication, and Right Supervision and Evaluation.
- **Accountability cannot be delegated.** The RN remains accountable for delegation decisions and patient outcomes even when tasks are performed by others.
- **Legal requirements for delegation vary by state.** Know your state's Nurse Practice Act and your facility's policies before delegating.

3.8 Practice Problems

Directions: Select the best answer for each question. Answers and rationales are provided in the Answer Key.

1. Which statement best describes the difference between delegation and assignment?

A. Delegation and assignment are the same thing and can be used interchangeably

B. Delegation involves transferring tasks that require nursing judgment to determine appropriateness; assignment involves distributing routine duties within scope of practice

C. Assignment requires more supervision than delegation

D. Only charge nurses can make assignments; any RN can delegate

2. According to the Five Rights of Delegation, which question should the nurse ask first when considering delegation?

A. "Is this person available to do this task?"

B. "Is this task appropriate to delegate?"

C. "What supervision will be required?"

D. "Have I documented this delegation?"

3. A nurse is delegating vital signs to a UAP. Which instruction demonstrates appropriate "Right Direction and Communication"?

A. "Check the vitals on the patient in 302 when you get a chance."

B. "Get vital signs on Mrs. Adams in 302. Report to me immediately if her blood pressure is below 90 systolic or above 180, or if her pulse is irregular. I need these within 20 minutes."

C. "Do the vitals on 302 like you usually do."

D. "The patient in 302 needs vitals—you know what to do."

4. A UAP tells the nurse, "I've never been trained to do blood glucose checks." What should the nurse do?

A. Delegate the task anyway because blood glucose checks are basic skills

B. Show the UAP how to do it once and then delegate the task

C. Not delegate this task to this UAP and either perform it or find someone who is trained

D. Report the UAP to management for incompetence

5. Which task is appropriate for an RN to delegate to a UAP?

A. Developing a care plan for a newly admitted patient

B. Administering oral medications to a stable patient

C. Assisting a stable patient with a bed bath

D. Performing initial patient teaching about a new diagnosis

6. A nurse delegates a task to a UAP. The UAP performs the task incorrectly, and the patient is harmed. Who is accountable?

A. Only the UAP, because they performed the task incorrectly

B. Only the nurse, because they delegated the task

C. Both the nurse and the UAP have accountability—the nurse for the delegation decision and the UAP for their actions

D. Neither, because it was an honest mistake

7. According to the Five Rights of Delegation, "Right Circumstance" refers to:

A. Whether the delegatee is competent to perform the task

B. Whether the patient's condition and setting are appropriate for delegation

C. Whether clear instructions have been provided

D. Whether appropriate follow-up has occurred

8. A nurse asks a UAP to obtain vital signs on a patient who is receiving a blood transfusion. The nurse instructs the UAP to report immediately if the patient develops fever, chills, or shortness of breath. This is an example of:

A. Inappropriate delegation because UAPs cannot care for patients receiving transfusions

B. Appropriate delegation with clear parameters for reporting

C. Assignment rather than delegation

D. Delegation that violates the Right Task principle

9. Which statement about delegation accountability is correct?

A. When a nurse delegates a task, accountability transfers to the delegatee

B. The nurse can delegate both responsibility and accountability

C. The nurse remains accountable for the delegation decision and patient outcome

D. Accountability is shared equally between the nurse and delegatee

10. A nurse is hesitant to delegate because "I can do it faster myself." What is the best response to this barrier?

A. This is a valid reason to avoid delegation

B. While it may be true initially, delegation develops team skills and improves long-term efficiency

C. Nurses should never delegate tasks they can do themselves

D. Speed is the most important factor in delegation decisions

11. Which factor would make delegation of vital signs to a UAP inappropriate?

A. The patient is stable with no changes in condition

B. The UAP has been trained and has demonstrated competence

C. The patient is showing signs of clinical deterioration and requires nursing assessment

D. The facility policy permits UAPs to obtain vital signs

12. A nurse from State A moves to State B and assumes delegation practices are the same. What is the potential problem with this assumption?

A. There is no problem; delegation rules are nationally standardized

B. State Nurse Practice Acts vary, and what is permitted in one state may be prohibited in another

C. Only facility policies matter, not state regulations

D. Delegation is never permitted when nurses relocate

13. The nurse receives a report that a UAP did not complete a delegated task. What should the nurse do first?

A. Report the UAP to the supervisor immediately

B. Complete the task and speak with the UAP about what happened

C. Document that the UAP is incompetent

D. Refuse to work with the UAP in the future

14. Which action demonstrates appropriate supervision after delegation?

A. Assuming the task was completed correctly and moving on to other duties

B. Following up to verify task completion and evaluating the outcome

C. Hovering over the delegatee and correcting every minor deviation

D. Waiting for the delegatee to report problems without checking in

15. A nurse needs to delegate a task but is unsure if the UAP is competent. What is the best action?

A. Delegate the task and monitor closely

B. Delegate the task with extra instructions

C. Verify the UAP's training and competency before delegating

D. Avoid delegation and perform all tasks personally

16. According to delegation principles, which task can NEVER be delegated by an RN?

A. Obtaining vital signs on stable patients

B. Assisting with activities of daily living

C. Performing initial patient assessment

D. Collecting routine urine specimens

17. A UAP says, "The patient in 305 seems different today." What should the nurse do?

A. Tell the UAP not to worry about things outside their scope

B. Thank the UAP and assess the patient promptly

C. Ask the UAP to document their concern

D. Ignore the comment because UAPs cannot assess patients

18. Which situation represents an appropriate reason for a delegatee to refuse a delegated task?

A. The delegatee does not like the task

B. The delegatee has not been trained to perform the task

C. The delegatee is busy with other assigned duties

D. The delegatee thinks the nurse should do it

19. What is the primary legal authority governing delegation in nursing practice?

A. Federal nursing laws

B. Hospital policies

C. State Nurse Practice Acts

D. American Nurses Association recommendations

20. A new graduate nurse is overwhelmed and afraid to delegate because of concerns about accountability. Which statement would be most helpful?

A. "You shouldn't delegate until you have more experience."

B. "Delegation is optional—just do everything yourself if you're uncomfortable."

C. "Using the Five Rights framework helps ensure safe delegation, and appropriate delegation is part of professional nursing practice."

D. "Don't worry about accountability—the facility will protect you."

End of Chapter 3 Practice Problems

CHAPTER 4

Scope of Practice

4.1 Learning Objectives

By the end of this chapter, you will be able to:

- Define scope of practice and explain its legal basis
- Differentiate the scopes of practice for RNs, LPNs/LVNs, and UAPs
- Identify tasks that can never be delegated
- Apply scope of practice knowledge to delegation decisions

4.2 Understanding Scope of Practice

Scope of practice is one of the most important concepts in nursing—and one of the most commonly misunderstood. Every delegation decision you make depends on understanding not just your own scope of practice, but also the scopes of practice of every team member you work with.

What Is Scope of Practice?

Scope of practice defines the activities that a healthcare professional is legally authorized to perform. It establishes the boundaries of what you can and cannot do based on your education, training, licensure, and competency.

Scope of practice is not a suggestion or a guideline—it is a legal boundary. Working outside your scope of practice can result in:

- Disciplinary action by the Board of Nursing
- Loss of licensure
- Civil liability (lawsuits)
- Criminal charges in extreme cases
- Termination of employment
- Patient harm

Sources of Scope of Practice

Scope of practice is determined by multiple overlapping sources:

State Nurse Practice Acts. Each state has a Nurse Practice Act (NPA) that defines what nurses can legally do in that state. The NPA establishes the legal scope of practice for RNs, LPNs/LVNs, and sometimes advanced practice nurses. This is the primary legal authority.

State Board of Nursing Rules and Regulations. Boards of Nursing issue rules that interpret and expand upon the Nurse Practice Act. These rules often provide more specific guidance about particular tasks or situations.

Facility Policies and Procedures. Healthcare facilities establish policies that may further define or limit scope of practice. Facility policies can be more restrictive than state law but cannot expand scope beyond what the law allows.

Professional Standards. Organizations like the American Nurses Association (ANA) publish standards of practice that describe expected competencies. While not legally binding, these standards influence how scope of practice is interpreted.

Job Descriptions. Your specific job description may limit your practice to certain activities, even if your license would permit broader practice.

Individual Competency. Even if something is within your legal scope, you should not perform it unless you have the knowledge and skill to do so safely. Scope of practice sets the outer boundary; competency determines what you can actually do within that boundary.

The Hierarchy of Authority

When these sources conflict, there is a hierarchy:

1. **State law (Nurse Practice Act)** — The absolute ceiling; nothing can exceed this
2. **Board of Nursing rules** — Interpret state law
3. **Facility policies** — Can restrict but not expand beyond law
4. **Job descriptions** — Can further limit within facility policies
5. **Individual competency** — Your personal limit within all of the above

Example: State law permits RNs to administer IV push medications. Your hospital's policy also permits this. However, your unit's orientation does not include IV push competency validation. Even though state law and hospital policy permit it, you should not administer IV push medications until you have demonstrated competency on your unit.

Scope of Practice Varies by State

One of the most important things to understand is that **scope of practice varies significantly from state to state**. What an LPN can do in one state may be prohibited in another. What requires physician supervision in one state may be independent practice in another.

If you relocate to a new state, work in a border region, or work via telehealth across state lines, you must verify the scope of practice rules for each state where you practice. Never assume that rules from one state apply to another.

4.3 RN Scope of Practice

The registered nurse has the broadest scope of practice among nursing personnel. RNs are educated and licensed to provide comprehensive nursing care, including complex assessment, planning, intervention, and evaluation.

Core RN Functions

The following activities are core RN functions that cannot be delegated:

Comprehensive Assessment. The RN performs the initial and ongoing comprehensive assessment of patients. This includes collecting health history, performing physical examination, identifying patient problems, and recognizing changes in condition. While others may collect data (like vital signs), the RN is responsible for interpreting that data and making clinical judgments.

Nursing Diagnosis. Based on assessment data, the RN identifies nursing diagnoses—clinical judgments about patient responses to health conditions. This requires the analytical and critical thinking skills that RN education provides.

Care Planning. The RN develops the plan of care, establishing priorities, setting goals, and selecting interventions. The RN may collaborate with the patient, family, and other healthcare providers, but the responsibility for the nursing care plan rests with the RN.

Implementation of Complex Interventions. While some interventions can be delegated, complex interventions requiring nursing judgment remain with the RN. This includes interventions that require ongoing assessment during performance, interventions with unpredictable outcomes, and interventions requiring modification based on patient response.

Evaluation. The RN evaluates patient progress toward goals and the effectiveness of interventions. This evaluation requires clinical judgment to determine whether the plan should continue, be modified, or be discontinued.

Patient Education. Initial and complex patient education is an RN responsibility. While reinforcement of teaching may be delegated, the RN is responsible for assessing learning needs, developing teaching plans, and evaluating learning outcomes.

Coordination of Care. The RN coordinates care across the healthcare team, communicates with providers, and ensures continuity of care.

RN Authority to Delegate

A key component of RN scope of practice is the authority to delegate. The RN:

- Determines what can be delegated
- Selects the appropriate person to receive delegation
- Communicates effectively about the delegated task
- Supervises the delegated task
- Evaluates outcomes

This authority comes with accountability. The RN cannot simply hand off tasks without regard for patient safety and appropriate supervision.

Variations in RN Scope

Even among RNs, scope of practice may vary based on:

Specialty Certification. Certified nurses in specialties like critical care (CCRN), oncology (OCN), or emergency nursing (CEN) may have additional competencies, though certification itself does not change legal scope.

Practice Setting. RNs in different settings (hospital, ambulatory care, home health, school nursing) may have different practical scopes based on available resources and supervision.

Advanced Practice. Advanced Practice Registered Nurses (APRNs) including Nurse Practitioners, Clinical Nurse Specialists, Nurse Midwives, and Nurse Anesthetists have expanded scopes that include activities like prescribing medications and diagnosing conditions. APRN scope is beyond the focus of this chapter but is governed by additional state regulations.

4.4 LPN/LVN Scope of Practice

Licensed Practical Nurses (LPNs), called Licensed Vocational Nurses (LVNs) in California and Texas, have a more focused scope of practice than RNs. LPNs provide care under the direction of an RN or physician.

LPN Education and Role

LPN programs are typically 12-18 months and prepare graduates for a technical, task-oriented role. LPNs are educated to:

- Collect data (but not perform comprehensive assessment)
- Contribute to care planning (but not develop the plan independently)
- Implement interventions within their scope
- Report findings to the RN
- Provide direct patient care in stable, predictable situations

What LPNs Can Typically Do

While specific permissions vary by state, LPNs commonly can:

- Obtain vital signs and report abnormalities
- Perform basic physical assessments on stable patients
- Administer oral, topical, subcutaneous, and intramuscular medications
- Perform wound care and dressing changes
- Insert urinary catheters
- Provide tracheostomy care and suctioning

- Administer enteral feedings
- Collect specimens
- Provide personal care and ADL assistance
- Document care provided
- Reinforce patient teaching (not initial teaching)

What LPNs Typically Cannot Do

Activities typically outside LPN scope include:

- Initial comprehensive assessment
- Developing nursing care plans
- Initial patient education
- Triage
- Receiving telephone orders (in many states)
- Administering IV push medications (in most states)
- Initiating blood transfusions (in most states)
- Caring for unstable patients without RN supervision

IV Therapy and LPNs

IV therapy is one of the most variable areas of LPN practice. Rules differ significantly by state:

- **Some states:** LPNs cannot perform any IV therapy
- **Some states:** LPNs can monitor existing IVs but not start them
- **Some states:** LPNs can start peripheral IVs and administer IV fluids
- **Some states:** LPNs can administer certain IV medications with additional certification
- **Few states:** LPNs can administer IV push medications

You must know your specific state's rules about LPN IV therapy. Never assume an LPN can or cannot perform IV-related tasks without verifying state regulations.

LPN Supervision Requirements

LPNs practice under the supervision of an RN or physician. The required level of supervision varies:

Direct supervision: The RN or physician is physically present and immediately available. This may be required for complex tasks or unstable patients.

Indirect supervision: The RN or physician is available by phone or can be present within a reasonable time. This is common for routine care of stable patients.

In some settings, like long-term care, LPNs may function with considerable autonomy for stable patients while an RN provides periodic oversight. In acute care, closer RN supervision is typical.

4.5 UAP Scope of Practice

Unlicensed Assistive Personnel (UAPs) include nursing assistants, patient care technicians, certified nursing assistants (CNAs), medical assistants, and other unlicensed workers who assist with patient care under nursing supervision.

UAP Education and Certification

UAP training varies widely:

Certified Nursing Assistants (CNAs) complete state-approved training programs (typically 75-120 hours) and pass a competency evaluation. CNAs are listed on a state registry. Federal law requires CNA certification for workers in Medicare/Medicaid-certified nursing facilities.

Patient Care Technicians (PCTs) may have additional training beyond CNA, such as phlebotomy, EKG, or basic laboratory skills. Training and certification requirements vary by employer.

Nursing Assistants without certification may work in some settings with on-the-job training, though this is increasingly uncommon.

Medical Assistants are trained for ambulatory settings and may perform clinical and administrative tasks. Their scope varies significantly by state.

What UAPs Can Typically Do

UAPs are trained to perform delegated tasks that:

- Are routine and repetitive
- Do not require nursing judgment during performance
- Have predictable outcomes
- Can be safely performed with the patient's current condition

Common UAP tasks include:

- Vital signs on stable patients
- Height and weight measurement
- Intake and output monitoring
- Blood glucose monitoring (with training, in many states)
- Bathing, grooming, and hygiene assistance
- Dressing assistance
- Feeding assistance (non-complex)

- Ambulation and mobility assistance
- Positioning and turning
- Bed making and linen changes
- Specimen collection (routine)
- Transport of stable patients
- Range of motion exercises
- Application of simple dressings (non-sterile)
- Stocking supplies

What UAPs Cannot Do

UAPs cannot perform tasks that require:

- Professional licensure
- Nursing judgment
- Assessment or interpretation of findings
- Sterile technique (in most settings)
- Medication administration (with limited exceptions)

Specifically, UAPs cannot:

- Perform assessments or interpret data
- Administer medications (except in specific training programs)
- Insert invasive devices (IVs, catheters)
- Provide patient education
- Take telephone orders
- Perform triage
- Make clinical decisions
- Provide care requiring ongoing nursing judgment

Medication Exceptions

In some states and settings, UAPs may administer medications with special training:

Medication Aides/Technicians. Some states credential medication aides who can administer certain medications (usually oral) in specific settings like long-term care or assisted living. Requirements vary significantly.

Insulin Administration. A few states permit trained UAPs to administer routine insulin injections to stable patients in specific settings.

School Settings. Some states permit trained school personnel to administer emergency medications like epinephrine auto-injectors or rescue inhalers.

These are exceptions, not the rule. In most acute care settings, UAPs do not administer medications. Always verify your state's specific regulations.

UAP Supervision

UAPs work under the direct supervision of licensed nurses. Key supervision principles:

- The RN is responsible for delegating appropriately
- The RN determines the level of supervision needed
- The UAP reports findings to the licensed nurse
- The UAP does not interpret findings or make clinical decisions
- The licensed nurse evaluates outcomes of delegated care

UAPs are not independent practitioners. They are extensions of the nursing team who perform delegated tasks to support patient care.

4.6 Tasks That Can Never Be Delegated

Certain nursing activities can never be delegated, regardless of the delegatee's training or experience. These tasks require the professional judgment, education, and accountability that only licensed nurses possess.

The Nursing Process

The core components of the nursing process are RN responsibilities:

Assessment. The initial comprehensive assessment and ongoing assessment of patient status require RN-level education and judgment. While UAPs may collect data (vital signs, intake/output), the interpretation and clinical judgment about that data is an RN function.

Diagnosis. Identifying nursing diagnoses requires analysis and clinical reasoning that only the RN is educated to perform.

Planning. Developing the nursing care plan, setting priorities, and selecting interventions require RN judgment. Others may contribute information, but the RN is responsible for the plan.

Evaluation. Determining whether goals have been met and whether the care plan should be modified requires RN-level clinical judgment.

Note: Implementation can be partially delegated, depending on the specific intervention.

Clinical Judgment Activities

Any activity requiring clinical judgment during its performance cannot be delegated:

- Interpreting assessment findings

- Recognizing changes in patient condition
- Making decisions about interventions
- Determining urgency or priority
- Modifying care based on patient response
- Evaluating treatment effectiveness

Communication With Providers

Professional communication requiring nursing judgment cannot be delegated:

- Receiving and transcribing telephone or verbal orders
- Providing clinical reports to physicians
- Notifying providers of changes in patient condition
- Participating in interdisciplinary rounds (representing nursing perspective)

Specific Tasks That Cannot Be Delegated

Triage. Determining the urgency of patient needs and prioritizing care requires RN assessment and judgment.

Initial Patient Education. Assessing learning needs, developing teaching plans, and providing initial education require RN skills. Reinforcement may be delegated.

Discharge Planning. Coordinating discharge and ensuring patients are prepared to manage their care requires RN assessment and planning.

Admission Assessment. The comprehensive admission assessment is an RN function.

Care of Unstable Patients. Patients who are unstable, unpredictable, or at high risk for deterioration require RN care. Delegation is only appropriate for stable patients.

Invasive Procedures Requiring Nursing Judgment. While some invasive procedures may be within LPN scope, any procedure requiring ongoing nursing judgment during performance remains with the RN.

4.7 Common Delegation Scenarios

The following table summarizes common tasks and their appropriateness for different team members. Remember that state laws and facility policies may differ from these general guidelines.

Delegation Decision Table

Task	RN	LPN/LVN	UAP	Notes
Initial comprehensive assessment	✓	RN only—cannot be delegated		
Focused assessment (stable patient)	✓	✓	LPN collects data; RN interprets	
Vital signs (stable patient)	✓	✓	✓	UAP reports; nurse interprets

Task	RN	LPN/LVN	UAP	Notes
Vital signs (unstable patient)	✓	✓	Requires licensed assessment	
Develop nursing care plan	✓	RN only		
Implement routine care plan	✓	✓	✓	Depending on specific task
Medication administration—oral	✓	✓	*	*Only trained medication aides in some states/settings
Medication administration—IM/SQ	✓	✓		
Medication administration—IV	✓	*	*State-dependent; many states limit LPN IV	
IV push medications	✓	*	*Few states permit LPN; requires additional training	
Blood transfusion initiation	✓	RN only in most states		
Blood transfusion monitoring	✓	✓	LPN can monitor once initiated	
Wound care—simple dressing	✓	✓	✓	Non-sterile, simple wounds
Wound care—complex/sterile	✓	✓	Requires sterile technique	
Wound assessment	✓	✓	UAP cannot assess wounds	
Urinary catheter insertion	✓	✓		
Urinary catheter care	✓	✓	✓	Routine care only
Tracheostomy suctioning	✓	✓	*	*Some states allow trained UAPs
Tracheostomy care	✓	✓		
Feeding—uncomplicated	✓	✓	✓	No aspiration risk
Feeding—aspiration risk	✓	✓	Requires licensed supervision	
Enteral tube feeding	✓	✓	*	*State/setting dependent
Blood glucose monitoring	✓	✓	✓	With training
Specimen collection—routine	✓	✓	✓	Clean catch, stool, etc.
Specimen collection—sterile	✓	✓	Catheter specimens, etc.	
Patient education—initial	✓	RN only		
Patient education—reinforcement	✓	✓	LPN reinforces RN teaching	
Discharge teaching	✓	RN only		
Receive telephone orders	✓	*	*Some states permit LPN	
Triage	✓	RN only		
Ambulation (stable patient)	✓	✓	✓	
ADL assistance	✓	✓	✓	
Positioning/turning	✓	✓	✓	
Intake/output measurement	✓	✓	✓	UAP measures; nurse evaluates
Documentation	✓	✓	✓	Each documents own care

Key Principles for Using This Table

1. **This is a general guide.** Always verify your state's Nurse Practice Act and your facility's policies.

2. **Consider the patient.** Even tasks that can generally be delegated may be inappropriate for a specific unstable patient.

3. **Consider the person.** Tasks should only be delegated to individuals who have demonstrated competency.

4. **State variations matter.** Especially for LPN IV therapy, medication aide programs, and UAP tasks—check your state.

5. **When in doubt, do not delegate.** If you are unsure whether delegation is appropriate, err on the side of caution.

4.8 Key Takeaways

- **Scope of practice is a legal boundary** defining what each healthcare professional can do. It is determined by state law, Board of Nursing rules, facility policies, job descriptions, and individual competency.
- **Scope of practice varies by state.** Never assume rules from one state apply to another. Verify regulations when you relocate or practice across state lines.
- **RNs have the broadest scope** and are responsible for assessment, diagnosis, planning, and evaluation. RNs have authority and accountability for delegation decisions.
- **LPNs/LVNs have a focused scope** and work under RN or physician supervision. LPN scope, especially for IV therapy, varies significantly by state.
- **UAPs perform delegated tasks** under licensed nurse supervision. They collect data but do not interpret it or make clinical decisions.
- **Some tasks can never be delegated:** initial assessment, nursing diagnosis, care planning, evaluation, triage, initial teaching, and any activity requiring nursing judgment during performance.

4.9 Practice Problems

Directions: Select the best answer for each question. Answers and rationales are provided in the Answer Key.

1. A new graduate nurse asks, "What determines my scope of practice?" Which response is most accurate?

A. Your scope is determined solely by your employer's job description

B. Your scope is determined primarily by your state's Nurse Practice Act, along with Board of Nursing rules, facility policies, and your competency

C. Your scope is the same in every state once you pass the NCLEX

D. Your scope is determined by what your preceptor tells you to do

2. An RN is making delegation decisions for the shift. Which task can ONLY be performed by the RN?

A. Obtaining vital signs on a stable post-operative patient

B. Performing the initial comprehensive assessment on a new admission

C. Administering oral medications to a stable patient

D. Ambulating a patient on the first day after hip replacement

3. An LPN asks the RN, "Can I give this IV push medication?" What should the RN do first?

A. Allow the LPN to give it because LPNs can give all medications

B. Check the state's Nurse Practice Act and facility policy regarding LPN IV push administration

C. Refuse because LPNs can never give IV medications

D. Delegate the task to a UAP instead

4. Which task is within the scope of practice for a UAP?

A. Assessing a patient's lung sounds

B. Determining whether a patient's pain medication is effective

C. Obtaining vital signs on a stable patient and reporting results to the nurse

D. Deciding which patient should be seen first

5. A nurse from Florida relocates to California. What should the nurse understand about scope of practice?

A. Scope of practice is federally regulated and identical in all states

B. Scope of practice may differ; the nurse must verify California regulations before practicing

C. The nurse's Florida license automatically determines California scope

D. Scope of practice only matters for advanced practice nurses

6. Which statement about LPN scope of practice is accurate?

A. LPNs can independently develop nursing care plans

B. LPNs work under the direction of an RN or physician

C. LPN scope of practice is identical in all states

D. LPNs can always administer IV push medications

7. An RN is supervising a UAP. Which action by the UAP requires the RN to intervene?

A. The UAP measures and records the patient's intake and output

B. The UAP reports that a patient's blood pressure is higher than usual

C. The UAP tells a patient that their blood pressure is "probably nothing to worry about"

D. The UAP assists a stable patient with ambulation

8. A patient requires discharge teaching about a new medication. Who should provide this teaching?

A. The UAP, because it frees the nurse for other tasks

B. The LPN, because medication teaching is within LPN scope

C. The RN, because initial patient education is an RN responsibility

D. Any available staff member with time

9. Which scenario demonstrates appropriate delegation based on scope of practice?

A. An RN asks a UAP to assess whether a patient's surgical wound is healing properly

B. An RN asks an LPN to administer oral medications to stable patients

C. An RN asks a UAP to determine which of two patients should receive pain medication first

D. An RN asks an LPN to develop the care plan for a newly admitted patient

10. A charge nurse is assigning patients. The unit has one RN, one LPN, and one UAP. Which assignment is most appropriate?

A. Assign the unstable patient with chest pain to the LPN

B. Assign the stable post-operative patient requiring routine care to the LPN

C. Assign all initial assessments to the UAP

D. Assign discharge teaching to the LPN

11. An LPN reports to the RN that a patient's condition has changed. What is the RN's responsibility?

A. Thank the LPN and document the report at the end of the shift

B. Tell the LPN to handle it independently

C. Assess the patient and determine if intervention is needed

D. Delegate the assessment to the UAP

12. Which activity can never be delegated to a UAP regardless of training?

A. Blood glucose monitoring

B. Vital sign measurement

C. Interpreting whether vital signs indicate patient deterioration

D. Assisting with patient ambulation

13. A nursing student asks why scope of practice matters. What is the best response?

A. "Scope of practice is just bureaucratic paperwork that doesn't affect patient care."

B. "Scope of practice protects patients by ensuring care is provided by qualified individuals, and protects your license by defining legal boundaries."

C. "Scope of practice only matters if someone files a lawsuit."

D. "Scope of practice can be ignored if you feel confident in your skills."

14. An RN is working in a state that permits LPNs to initiate peripheral IVs. The RN's facility policy prohibits LPNs from starting IVs. What should guide the RN's delegation decision?

A. Follow state law and allow the LPN to start IVs

B. Follow facility policy and do not delegate IV starts to the LPN

C. Let the LPN decide based on their comfort level

D. Check with the patient about their preference

15. A UAP has completed additional training as a phlebotomist. Which statement about this UAP's scope is correct?

A. The UAP can now perform any task an LPN can perform

B. The UAP can perform phlebotomy as trained, but other scope limitations remain unchanged

C. Additional training automatically expands all scope of practice boundaries

D. Training does not affect scope of practice in any way

16. Which task is most appropriate for an RN to delegate to an LPN caring for stable patients?

A. Admitting a new patient and completing the initial assessment

B. Administering prescribed oral and intramuscular medications

C. Evaluating whether the patient has met discharge criteria

D. Triaging phone calls from patients

17. A UAP notices that a patient seems confused, which is different from earlier in the shift. What should the UAP do?

A. Document the finding and continue with other tasks

B. Determine what is causing the confusion

C. Report the observation to the licensed nurse immediately

D. Administer PRN medication for agitation

18. An RN delegates vital signs for a stable patient to a UAP. The UAP reports back that the blood pressure was 88/56. What should the RN do?

A. Thank the UAP and document the finding for the provider to review later

B. Ask the UAP what they think is causing the low blood pressure

C. Assess the patient personally because interpretation of findings is an RN responsibility

D. Delegate the assessment to the LPN

19. Which statement about triage is correct?

A. Triage can be delegated to experienced LPNs

B. Triage can be performed by UAPs with additional training

C. Triage requires nursing judgment and can only be performed by an RN

D. Triage is an administrative task that anyone can perform

20. A new RN is unsure whether a task can be delegated to an LPN. What is the best action?

A. Delegate the task and learn from any problems that occur

B. Refuse to delegate anything to LPNs to avoid risk

C. Check the state Nurse Practice Act, Board of Nursing rules, and facility policy before delegating

D. Ask the LPN if they are comfortable doing the task

End of Chapter 4 Practice Problems

CHAPTER 5

Making Safe Assignments

5.1 Learning Objectives

By the end of this chapter, you will be able to:

- Describe the principles of safe patient assignment
- Identify factors that influence assignment decisions
- Explain the charge nurse's role in making assignments
- Recognize when and how to address unsafe assignments

5.2 Principles of Safe Assignment

While delegation involves transferring specific tasks, assignment refers to the distribution of work among team members—determining which nurse cares for which patients and which support staff works with which nurses. Safe assignment is foundational to safe patient care.

What Is Assignment?

Assignment is the distribution of work that each staff member is responsible for during a given shift. Unlike delegation, which involves transferring responsibility for specific tasks, assignment involves allocating overall responsibility for patient care to individuals for whom that care is within their scope of practice and job expectations.

When the charge nurse says, "You have rooms 401-404 tonight," that is an assignment. When you ask the UAP to obtain vital signs on your patients, that is delegation.

The Goal of Safe Assignment

The goal of safe assignment is to match patient needs with staff competencies in a way that ensures:

- **Patient safety** — Patients receive care from qualified individuals
- **Quality care** — Staff can meet patient needs effectively
- **Reasonable workload** — No staff member is dangerously overloaded
- **Appropriate supervision** — Less experienced staff have adequate support
- **Continuity of care** — When possible, patients have consistent caregivers

Who Makes Assignments?

Assignment responsibility varies by setting:

Charge Nurses typically make shift assignments in acute care settings. They consider patient acuity, staff competencies, and unit needs when distributing the workload.

Nurse Managers may make assignments or oversee the assignment process, especially for scheduling and longer-term staffing decisions.

Staff Nurses may participate in assignment decisions, particularly in self-scheduling units or when adjustments are needed during a shift.

House Supervisors often coordinate assignments across units, especially when floating staff or managing house-wide staffing shortages.

Assignment vs. Delegation: A Critical Distinction

Understanding the difference between assignment and delegation is essential:

Aspect	Assignment	Delegation
What it involves	Distributing overall patient care responsibility	Transferring specific tasks
Who receives it	Licensed personnel working within their scope	Anyone qualified for the specific task
Accountability	The assigned nurse is accountable for their patients	The delegating nurse retains accountability
Frequency	Typically once per shift	Throughout the shift as needed
Decision maker	Usually charge nurse or manager	Individual RN for their patients

Example: The charge nurse assigns an LPN to care for four stable medical patients (assignment). During the shift, the RN covering the unit asks the LPN to obtain a set of vital signs on one of the RN's patients who is showing signs of change (delegation).

5.3 Factors Influencing Assignments

Making safe assignments requires balancing multiple factors. No formula works for every situation—clinical judgment is essential.

Patient Factors

Acuity and Stability. How sick are the patients? Unstable patients require more nursing time and expertise. A nurse with four unstable patients may be dangerously overloaded, while another nurse might safely manage six stable patients.

Complexity of Care. What interventions do patients require? Complex wound care, multiple IV medications, frequent monitoring, or specialized equipment all increase the time and skill required.

Predictability. Are patient conditions expected to remain stable, or is deterioration likely? Post-operative patients in the first hours after surgery need closer monitoring than those on post-op day three.

Special Needs. Do patients have needs requiring specific competencies? Examples include patients on ventilators, those receiving chemotherapy, patients with tracheostomies, or those requiring specialized monitoring.

Isolation Requirements. Patients in isolation require additional time for donning and doffing PPE and may need to be grouped to minimize staff exposure.

Psychosocial Needs. Patients with high anxiety, difficult family situations, end-of-life care needs, or behavioral health concerns require additional nursing time.

Staff Factors

Licensure and Scope. What is each staff member legally permitted to do? RNs, LPNs, and UAPs have different scopes that must be matched to patient needs.

Competency and Experience. Beyond licensure, what can each person actually do well? A new graduate RN and a 20-year veteran have different capabilities even with the same license.

Specialty Training. Does the nurse have certifications or training relevant to specific patient populations? Examples include chemotherapy administration, cardiac monitoring interpretation, or pediatric expertise.

Familiarity with Patients. Has the nurse cared for these patients before? Continuity of care improves outcomes and efficiency.

Familiarity with Unit. Is the nurse regularly assigned to this unit or floating from elsewhere? Floating staff may need modified assignments.

Physical and Emotional Status. Is the staff member dealing with fatigue, illness, or personal stress that might affect performance? While this is sensitive, patient safety must come first.

Unit and System Factors

Total Census and Acuity. How many patients are on the unit, and what is the overall acuity level? High census with high acuity strains all resources.

Staffing Levels. How many staff members are available? Shortages require creative problem-solving and may necessitate escalation.

Admissions, Discharges, Transfers. Units with high turnover require additional time for admission assessments, discharge teaching, and transfer coordination.

Available Resources. What support is available? Adequate UAP support, available respiratory therapists, accessible providers, and functioning equipment all affect what nurses can manage.

Geographic Layout. How are rooms arranged? A nurse with patients scattered across the unit spends more time walking than one with clustered patients.

Time of Shift. Day shift typically has more scheduled activities (procedures, therapies, discharges); night shift may have fewer resources but also fewer planned activities.

Balancing Competing Factors

Assignment decisions often involve trade-offs:

- The most experienced nurse might be needed for the sickest patient, but that leaves less experienced nurses without a strong resource
- Continuity of care is valuable, but sometimes a fresh perspective or different skill set is needed
- Clustering assignments geographically is efficient, but patient needs must still drive decisions
- New staff need learning opportunities, but patient safety cannot be compromised for education

There is no perfect formula. Good assignment decisions require clinical judgment, knowledge of staff capabilities, and ongoing reassessment.

5.4 The Charge Nurse Role

The charge nurse plays a pivotal role in patient safety through assignment decisions and shift coordination. Understanding this role helps all nurses work more effectively.

Charge Nurse Responsibilities

Making Initial Assignments. The charge nurse typically creates the initial assignment at the beginning of each shift, considering all the factors discussed above.

Adjusting Assignments. Conditions change. Admissions arrive, patients deteriorate, staff members become ill. The charge nurse must be prepared to adjust assignments throughout the shift.

Coordinating Admissions. When new patients arrive, the charge nurse determines who will receive them, balancing current workloads and matching patient needs with nurse capabilities.

Serving as a Resource. Charge nurses often function as clinical resources, helping staff troubleshoot problems, answering questions, and providing support during difficult situations.

Escalating Concerns. When unit-level resources are insufficient, the charge nurse escalates to house supervisors, nurse managers, or administrators.

Communicating with Other Departments. The charge nurse often coordinates with other units, departments, and services regarding patient flow and resource needs.

What Makes a Good Assignment?

A good assignment:

- Matches patient acuity and needs with nurse competency and experience
- Distributes workload equitably (not necessarily equally—equity considers difficulty, not just numbers)
- Provides appropriate supervision for less experienced staff
- Maintains continuity of care when beneficial and possible

- Clusters patients geographically when patient needs allow
- Anticipates likely changes (expected admissions, potential discharges, patients who may deteriorate)
- Considers staff requests and preferences when patient safety allows

Supporting the Charge Nurse

Staff nurses can support effective assignments by:

- Communicating honestly about their competencies and limitations
- Reporting changes in patient condition promptly
- Offering to help colleagues who are struggling
- Raising concerns about assignments constructively
- Providing handoff information that accurately reflects patient acuity
- Being flexible when unit needs require adjustment

When You Disagree with an Assignment

If you believe an assignment is unsafe:

1. **Speak with the charge nurse privately.** Explain your specific concerns—what about this assignment creates risk?

2. **Be specific about the problem.** "I'm concerned" is less helpful than "I have three patients requiring q1h neuro checks, and Mr. Jones needs continuous monitoring during his transfusion."

3. **Propose solutions.** Can patients be redistributed? Can you get additional support? Is there a specific task that could be delegated or reassigned?

4. **Escalate if necessary.** If concerns are not resolved, escalate to the house supervisor or nurse manager.

5. **Document your concerns.** If you must accept an assignment you believe is unsafe, document your concerns through appropriate channels.

6. **Do not abandon patients.** Even if you believe an assignment is unsafe, refusing to care for patients who have already been assigned to you constitutes patient abandonment. Work within the system to address concerns while continuing to provide care.

5.5 Floating to Other Units

Floating—being reassigned to work on a unit other than your home unit—is a common practice for managing staffing needs. It also raises significant safety considerations.

Why Floating Occurs

Hospitals use floating to balance staffing across units when:

- One unit has more staff than needed while another is short
- Census fluctuates unpredictably
- Call-ins or illness create unexpected shortages
- High-acuity situations require additional support

Challenges of Floating

Floating creates challenges for both the floating nurse and the receiving unit:

Unfamiliar Environment. The floating nurse does not know where supplies are located, how the unit operates, or what resources are available.

Unfamiliar Patient Population. A medical-surgical nurse floating to a cardiac unit may be unfamiliar with specific cardiac medications, monitoring, or post-procedure care.

Unfamiliar Staff. The floating nurse does not know the capabilities of the unit's staff or who to ask for help.

Reduced Efficiency. Even experienced nurses work more slowly in unfamiliar settings.

Psychological Stress. Floating can be stressful, affecting confidence and performance.

Rights and Responsibilities When Floating

You Have the Right To:

- Receive an orientation to the unit (location of supplies, emergency equipment, key policies)
- Receive an assignment appropriate to your competencies
- Decline tasks outside your scope of practice or competency
- Access resources and support from unit staff
- Escalate concerns about unsafe assignments

You Have the Responsibility To:

- Communicate honestly about your competencies and limitations
- Ask for help when needed
- Follow unit policies and procedures
- Provide safe care within your capabilities
- Be flexible and professional despite the challenges

Safe Floating Practices

For the Floating Nurse:

- Immediately communicate your background and any limitations: "I'm a med-surg nurse. I'm not comfortable with cardiac drips or interpreting telemetry."

- Ask for orientation to essential locations: code cart, medication room, supply room, documentation system
- Request a resource person you can go to with questions
- Accept an assignment appropriate to your skills—stable patients with needs similar to those you typically manage
- Ask for help early rather than waiting until you are overwhelmed
- Document any concerns about the assignment

For the Receiving Unit:

- Provide orientation to the unit layout and essential procedures
- Assign patients whose needs match the floating nurse's competencies
- Identify a resource person for questions
- Check in periodically to ensure the floating nurse is managing
- Avoid assigning the most complex or unstable patients to floating staff

When Floating Is Inappropriate

You may legitimately decline or raise concerns about floating when:

- You lack the basic competencies required for the unit's patient population
- The receiving unit is asking you to perform tasks outside your scope
- You have not been oriented to essential equipment or procedures
- No appropriate resource support is available
- Patient safety would be compromised

However, floating within your competency is a reasonable expectation in most employment agreements. "I don't want to" or "I don't like that unit" are not legitimate reasons to refuse floating.

5.6 Refusing an Unsafe Assignment

There may be times when an assignment is so unsafe that you cannot accept it. This is a serious step with significant implications.

What Constitutes an Unsafe Assignment?

An assignment may be unsafe when:

- **Patient needs exceed nurse competencies.** You are assigned patients whose care requires knowledge or skills you do not possess.
- **Workload is unmanageable.** The number or acuity of patients makes it impossible to provide safe care.
- **Required supervision is unavailable.** An inexperienced nurse is left without adequate support.

- **Required resources are unavailable.** Essential equipment, medications, or support staff are not available.
- **Nurse impairment.** Illness, fatigue, or other factors make the nurse unable to perform safely.

Steps to Address Unsafe Assignments

1. **Identify the specific safety concern.** What exactly makes this assignment unsafe? Be concrete.

2. **Communicate with the charge nurse.** Express your concerns professionally and specifically. Propose alternatives if possible.

3. **Seek resolution at the unit level.** Can the assignment be modified? Can you receive additional support? Can tasks be redistributed?

4. **Escalate if unit-level resolution fails.** Contact the house supervisor, nurse manager, or nursing administrator.

5. **Document your concerns.** Complete any required documentation, such as an assignment-despite-objection (ADO) form or unsafe staffing report.

6. **Follow chain of command.** Continue escalating through the organizational hierarchy if needed.

7. **Consider professional resources.** Your state nurses association may have resources for addressing unsafe staffing.

Assignment Despite Objection (ADO)

Many facilities have a formal process for documenting when a nurse accepts an assignment they believe is unsafe. This assignment-despite-objection or protest-of-assignment documentation:

- Creates a record that you raised concerns
- May protect you legally by demonstrating you recognized risks
- Provides data that may support staffing improvements
- Should describe specific safety concerns, not general complaints

Using ADO documentation does not relieve you of responsibility to provide safe care—it documents that you raised concerns while continuing to meet your professional obligations.

What You Cannot Do

You cannot abandon patients. Once you have accepted responsibility for patients, you cannot simply leave them without care. Abandonment has serious legal and professional consequences.

You cannot refuse to work your scheduled shift without consequences, unless safety concerns meet very specific criteria and you follow proper procedures.

You cannot refuse a reasonable assignment simply because it is difficult, undesirable, or inconvenient.

Protecting Yourself Professionally

To protect yourself when facing difficult assignment situations:

- **Know your facility's policies** on staffing, floating, and assignment objection procedures
- **Document concerns** through appropriate channels
- **Communicate professionally** — how you raise concerns matters
- **Provide the best care possible** within the circumstances while working to change them
- **Know your state's safe staffing resources** — some states have specific staffing ratios or reporting mechanisms
- **Maintain records** of any incidents related to staffing concerns
- **Engage in staffing committees or councils** to address systemic issues

5.7 Assignment vs. Delegation Review

Because assignment and delegation are frequently confused, let's review the key distinctions:

Assignment

- **Definition:** Distribution of overall responsibility for patient care to nursing personnel
- **Who makes it:** Charge nurse, nurse manager, or supervisor
- **Who receives it:** Licensed nurses (RNs, LPNs) for patient care responsibility
- **Scope consideration:** The assigned nurse must be able to work within their scope for all assigned patients' needs
- **Accountability:** The assigned nurse is accountable for their assigned patients
- **Frequency:** Typically once per shift with adjustments as needed
- **Example:** "You have patients in rooms 201-204 tonight."

Delegation

- **Definition:** Transferring responsibility for performing a specific task while retaining accountability
- **Who makes it:** The RN responsible for the patient
- **Who receives it:** Anyone competent to perform the specific task (LPN, UAP)
- **Scope consideration:** The specific task must be within the delegatee's scope and competency
- **Accountability:** The delegating RN retains accountability for the delegation decision and outcome
- **Frequency:** Throughout the shift as patient care needs arise
- **Example:** "Please get vital signs on Mrs. Smith and report back to me."

How They Work Together

Assignment and delegation work together in practice:

1. The charge nurse **assigns** the RN to care for four patients

2. The RN **assesses** those patients and determines care needs

3. The RN **delegates** specific tasks to the UAP working with them

4. The RN **supervises** and **evaluates** the delegated tasks

5. The RN remains **accountable** for the care of assigned patients

Common Errors

Error: Treating delegation as assignment

"I assigned the UAP to do vitals on all my patients."

Problem: Delegation requires specific instructions and supervision for each delegated task, not a blanket "assignment."

Error: Failing to adjust assignments when conditions change

"I was assigned these patients at 7am; I can't take another admission."

Problem: Assignments must be fluid enough to accommodate changing unit needs.

Error: Accepting assignment of patients whose needs exceed your competency

"I've never cared for a ventilator patient, but the charge nurse assigned me one."

Problem: You must communicate limitations before accepting—not after something goes wrong.

Error: Delegating tasks that require nursing judgment

"I delegated the patient assessment to the LPN so I could focus on my other patients."

Problem: Initial assessment cannot be delegated; it requires RN-level judgment.

5.8 Key Takeaways

- **Assignment distributes overall patient care responsibility** to nursing personnel; delegation transfers specific tasks. They are related but distinct concepts.
- **Safe assignments match patient needs with staff competencies**, considering acuity, complexity, staff experience, and available resources.
- **The charge nurse plays a critical role** in making initial assignments, adjusting throughout the shift, coordinating admissions, and escalating concerns when needed.
- **When floating**, communicate your competencies and limitations, request appropriate orientation and assignment, and ask for help when needed.

- **Unsafe assignments should be addressed** through proper channels—communicate with the charge nurse, escalate as needed, document concerns, but do not abandon patients.
- **Know your facility's policies** on staffing, floating, and assignment objection, and use appropriate processes to address concerns.

5.9 Practice Problems

Directions: Select the best answer for each question. Answers and rationales are provided in the Answer Key.

1. Which statement best describes the difference between assignment and delegation?

A. Assignment and delegation are the same thing

B. Assignment distributes overall patient care responsibility; delegation transfers specific tasks

C. Delegation is done by charge nurses; assignment is done by staff nurses

D. Assignment involves UAPs; delegation involves only licensed nurses

2. The charge nurse is making assignments. Which factor is MOST important to consider first?

A. Nurse preferences for certain patient types

B. Geographic location of patient rooms

C. Matching patient acuity and needs with nurse competency

D. Ensuring equal numbers of patients per nurse

3. An RN receives an assignment of five patients including one who is intubated and on a ventilator. The RN has never cared for a ventilator patient. What should the RN do?

A. Accept the assignment and learn as they go

B. Refuse to come to work

C. Communicate this limitation to the charge nurse before accepting the assignment

D. Delegate ventilator care to the respiratory therapist

4. A nurse is asked to float to an oncology unit. The nurse works on a medical-surgical unit and has no chemotherapy training. Which action is most appropriate?

A. Refuse to float because the units are different

B. Accept the float but request an assignment that does not include chemotherapy administration

C. Administer chemotherapy after reading the procedure manual

D. Call in sick to avoid the float

5. Which patient would be MOST appropriate to assign to a new graduate nurse on orientation?

A. A patient with unstable angina requiring frequent nitroglycerin titration

B. A stable post-operative patient on day two after knee replacement

C. A patient receiving a blood transfusion for the first time

D. A patient with a new tracheostomy requiring frequent suctioning

6. The charge nurse assigns an LPN to four patients. During the shift, one patient becomes unstable with dropping blood pressure and altered mental status. What should happen?

A. The LPN should continue caring for the patient since they were assigned

B. The LPN should call the physician independently

C. An RN should assume care of the unstable patient or provide direct supervision

D. The UAP should be assigned to monitor the patient

7. A nurse believes their assignment is unsafe due to high acuity and inadequate staffing. After discussing with the charge nurse without resolution, what should the nurse do next?

A. Refuse to work and go home

B. Escalate to the house supervisor or nurse manager

C. Post concerns on social media

D. Simply do their best without documenting concerns

8. Which is an example of assignment rather than delegation?

A. The RN asks the UAP to obtain vital signs on a patient

B. The charge nurse distributes patient care responsibilities to nurses at shift start

C. The RN asks the LPN to reinforce discharge teaching

D. The RN directs the UAP to assist a patient with ambulation

9. A float nurse arrives on an unfamiliar unit. Which action by the receiving unit demonstrates best practice?

A. Assign the float nurse the most complex patients because they need experienced nurses

B. Assume the float nurse knows what to do and assign patients without orientation

C. Provide unit orientation and assign patients matching the float nurse's competencies

D. Tell the float nurse to figure things out on their own

10. An RN has concerns about an assignment but is told there are no other options. The RN should:

A. Abandon the patients and leave the unit

B. Accept the assignment, document concerns through proper channels, and provide the best care possible

C. Refuse to care for any patients until concerns are addressed

D. Ignore the concerns and hope nothing goes wrong

11. A charge nurse is making assignments and notices one RN will have three patients while another will have six. This is:

A. Always unfair and should never occur

B. Potentially appropriate if the three patients have higher acuity or complexity

C. Evidence of poor charge nurse skills

D. A violation of nursing regulations

12. Which situation would be an appropriate reason to refuse a float assignment?

A. You prefer working on your home unit

B. The float unit requires competencies you do not possess and no appropriate assignment is available

C. You floated last week and think it is someone else's turn

D. The float unit is busy and you want an easier shift

13. An experienced nurse notices that a new graduate on the unit appears overwhelmed with their assignment. What is the most appropriate action?

A. Ignore it—the new graduate needs to learn to manage independently

B. Report the new graduate to the manager for incompetence

C. Offer assistance and notify the charge nurse that the assignment may need adjustment

D. Take over all of the new graduate's patients

14. What is the primary purpose of assignment-despite-objection (ADO) documentation?

A. To get the charge nurse in trouble

B. To avoid having to care for difficult patients

C. To create a record of safety concerns while continuing to meet professional obligations

D. To ensure you won't be assigned difficult patients in the future

15. The charge nurse receives report that a new admission is coming from the ED. Which factors should the charge nurse consider when deciding who receives this patient? (Select the best answer.)

A. Which nurse has the lightest workload and competencies matching the patient's needs

B. Whose turn it is to receive an admission

C. Which nurse has been complaining the least

D. Which nurse is closest to the room where the patient will be placed

16. An LPN is assigned to care for a patient who needs initial discharge teaching about a new diabetes diagnosis. What should the LPN do?

A. Provide the teaching since the LPN was assigned to the patient

B. Ask the UAP to provide the teaching

C. Notify the RN that initial teaching is needed, as this is outside LPN scope

D. Tell the patient to look up information online

17. A nurse from the ICU is floated to a medical-surgical unit. Which assignment would be most appropriate for this nurse?

A. The most complex patients on the unit, since ICU nurses handle complex cases

B. An assignment similar to what med-surg nurses typically receive

C. Only patients who might need to transfer to ICU

D. No patient assignment—the ICU nurse should just help with tasks

18. Which statement about patient abandonment is correct?

A. Refusing an unsafe assignment before accepting it constitutes abandonment

B. Once you accept responsibility for patients, leaving without arranging coverage constitutes abandonment

C. Documenting an assignment-despite-objection constitutes abandonment

D. Escalating concerns to a supervisor constitutes abandonment

19. A charge nurse asks a staff nurse to take an additional admission, making their total patient count seven. The staff nurse feels this is unsafe. What is the best initial response?

A. "I refuse—that's too many patients."

B. "Absolutely, I can handle anything."

C. "I have concerns about safely managing seven patients given their current acuity. Can we discuss options?"

D. "Fine, but when something goes wrong it's your fault."

20. What is the most important principle guiding all assignment and floating decisions?

A. Staff satisfaction

B. Patient safety

C. Cost efficiency

D. Equal workload distribution

End of Chapter 5 Practice Problems

CHAPTER 6

Supervision and Communication

6.1 Learning Objectives

By the end of this chapter, you will be able to:

- Differentiate between levels of supervision and select the appropriate level
- Demonstrate effective communication techniques for delegation
- Apply the SBAR framework to delegation and clinical communication
- Describe appropriate follow-up and feedback after delegation

6.2 Levels of Supervision

Supervision is a critical component of safe delegation. The level of supervision required depends on the task, the patient, and the competency of the person performing the task. Selecting the appropriate level of supervision is part of the "Right Supervision" in the Five Rights of Delegation.

What Is Supervision?

Supervision is the provision of guidance, oversight, and evaluation by a qualified nurse for the accomplishment of a nursing task. Supervision includes:

- Initial direction and periodic inspection of the task
- Availability for guidance and assistance
- Evaluation of the outcome
- Follow-up and feedback

Supervision does not mean hovering over someone constantly. It means being appropriately available and attentive given the circumstances.

Levels of Supervision

The NCSBN describes supervision along a continuum from most intensive to least intensive:

Direct Supervision. The supervising nurse is physically present, observing the task as it is performed. Direct supervision is appropriate when:

- The delegatee is performing a task for the first time
- The delegatee is new to the unit or organization

- The task is complex or high-risk
- The patient is unstable or unpredictable
- The delegatee has expressed uncertainty about the task
- Organizational policy requires direct supervision for this task

Example: An RN directly supervises a new UAP performing blood glucose monitoring for the first time on the unit, observing technique and providing real-time feedback.

Indirect Supervision. The supervising nurse is not physically present but is immediately available for guidance. The nurse provides initial direction and is accessible for questions, checks progress periodically, and evaluates outcomes. Indirect supervision is appropriate when:

- The delegatee is competent and experienced with the task
- The task is routine and predictable
- The patient is stable
- The delegatee knows when and how to seek help
- Communication systems are in place for the delegatee to reach the nurse

Example: An RN delegates vital signs on four stable patients to an experienced UAP, asks to be notified of any abnormal values, and checks the results when completed.

Available Supervision. The supervising nurse is available for consultation but may not be on-site. This level is less common in acute care but may occur in some settings such as home health or community nursing where RNs supervise care provided by others at different locations.

Selecting the Appropriate Level

To determine the appropriate level of supervision, consider:

Task Factors

- How complex is the task?
- What are the risks if performed incorrectly?
- How predictable is the expected outcome?
- Does organizational policy specify a supervision level?

Patient Factors

- How stable is the patient?
- Are there factors that could cause unexpected changes?
- What would be the consequences of a problem?

Delegatee Factors

- How experienced is this person with this task?

- Have they demonstrated competency?
- Do they know when to ask for help?
- How comfortable and confident are they?

Environmental Factors

- What communication systems are available?
- How quickly can you respond if needed?
- What other resources are available?

Adjusting Supervision Over Time

Supervision is not static. As a delegatee demonstrates competence, the level of supervision can decrease:

1. **Initial phase:** Direct supervision while competency is established
2. **Developing phase:** Close indirect supervision with frequent check-ins
3. **Competent phase:** Standard indirect supervision with periodic follow-up
4. **Expert phase:** Minimal supervision—trusting the delegatee to perform and report appropriately

However, supervision should increase if:

- Patient condition changes
- The delegatee encounters an unfamiliar situation
- Problems or errors occur
- The delegatee requests additional support

6.3 Effective Delegation Communication

Communication is where delegation most often fails. Even when the right task is delegated to the right person in the right circumstance, poor communication can lead to errors, omissions, and patient harm. Effective delegation communication is a skill that must be learned and practiced.

Elements of Clear Delegation Communication

Every delegation should include:

1. The Specific Task

Be precise about what you are asking the person to do. Vague requests lead to misunderstandings.

- *Poor:* "Check on the patient in 302."
- *Better:* "Obtain a full set of vital signs on Mrs. Johnson in 302."

2. The Specific Patient

Always identify the patient by name and room number. Never assume the delegatee knows which patient you mean.

- *Poor:* "Get vitals on my new admission."
- *Better:* "Obtain vital signs on Mr. Williams in 308—he's my new admission from the ED."

3. The Timeline

When does the task need to be completed? Be specific.

- *Poor:* "When you get a chance."
- *Better:* "I need these vital signs within the next 30 minutes, before I call the physician."

4. Expected Findings

What is normal for this patient? What should the delegatee expect to find?

- *Poor:* "Let me know if anything is wrong."
- *Better:* "His blood pressure has been running 130-140 systolic. His normal heart rate is 70s-80s."

5. Reportable Conditions

What findings require immediate notification? Be specific about parameters.

- *Poor:* "Tell me if anything is abnormal."
- *Better:* "Report to me immediately if BP is below 100 or above 160 systolic, heart rate below 60 or above 100, or oxygen saturation below 92%."

6. When to Report Back

When do you expect to hear the results?

- *Poor:* (no mention of reporting)
- *Better:* "Come find me as soon as you have the results, or within 30 minutes, whichever comes first."

7. Opportunity for Questions

Always give the delegatee a chance to ask questions or seek clarification.

- "Do you have any questions?"
- "Does this make sense?"
- "Is there anything you're unsure about?"

The Two-Challenge Rule

If a delegatee has concerns about a delegated task, they should voice those concerns. Similarly, if you delegate something and the delegatee seems hesitant or uncertain, pay attention. The "two-challenge rule" from crew resource management suggests that concerns should be stated at least twice if the initial concern is not acknowledged.

For delegatees: If you are concerned about a task, speak up clearly. If your concern is dismissed, state it again more assertively.

For nurses delegating: If a delegatee expresses concern or hesitation, listen carefully. They may be aware of something you are not.

Closed-Loop Communication

Closed-loop communication ensures that messages are received and understood correctly. The process works like this:

1. **Sender delivers message:** "Please get vital signs on Mr. Williams in 308 and report back within 30 minutes."

2. **Receiver acknowledges and repeats back:** "I'll get vital signs on Mr. Williams in 308 and report back to you within 30 minutes."

3. **Sender confirms or corrects:** "That's correct" or "Actually, I need them within 15 minutes because the physician is calling back."

This simple technique dramatically reduces miscommunication.

Barriers to Effective Communication

Be aware of common barriers:

Interruptions and Distractions. Busy units are noisy and chaotic. Find a moment to communicate clearly rather than shouting instructions while walking past.

Assumptions. Never assume the delegatee knows what you mean. Be explicit.

Hierarchy and Intimidation. Some delegatees may be reluctant to ask questions or raise concerns. Create an environment where questions are welcomed.

Language Barriers. If there are language differences, speak clearly, avoid jargon, and verify understanding.

Incomplete Handoffs. Rushed communication leads to missing information. Take the time to communicate completely.

6.4 SBAR Communication Framework

SBAR (Situation, Background, Assessment, Recommendation) is a structured communication framework that improves clarity and completeness in clinical communication. Originally developed for high-risk industries like aviation and nuclear power, SBAR has been widely adopted in healthcare.

The SBAR Components

S – Situation

What is happening right now? State the current situation concisely.

- Who is the patient?
- What is the immediate issue?
- Why are you communicating?

Example: "I'm calling about Mrs. Rodriguez in 405. She's complaining of sudden onset chest pain."

B – Background

What is the relevant clinical background? Provide context that helps the listener understand the situation.

- Relevant diagnosis and history
- Recent changes or procedures
- Current treatment

Example: "She's a 68-year-old admitted yesterday with COPD exacerbation. She has a history of hypertension and diabetes. No cardiac history. She's been stable until now."

A – Assessment

What do you think is going on? Share your clinical assessment.

- What are the vital signs?
- What have you observed?
- What do you think the problem might be?

Example: "Her vitals are: BP 158/94, heart rate 102, respirations 22, O2 sat 94% on 2 liters. She's diaphoretic and anxious. I'm concerned this could be cardiac."

R – Recommendation

What do you think should happen? Make a specific request or recommendation.

- What do you need from the listener?
- What action do you recommend?

Example: "I think she needs an EKG and cardiac workup. Can you come evaluate her now?"

Using SBAR in Delegation

While SBAR is often used for nurse-to-physician communication, it can also structure delegation communication:

When delegating to UAP:

- **S:** "I need you to get vital signs on Mr. Chen in 412."
- **B:** "He's post-op day one from hip surgery, on blood thinners, and has been slightly hypotensive."
- **A:** "I'm monitoring him closely because of his bleeding risk."

- **R:** "Get vital signs now and report back immediately. Tell me right away if BP is below 100 systolic or heart rate over 100."

When UAP reports back:

The UAP can use a modified SBAR:

- **S:** "I have the vital signs on Mr. Chen."
- **B:** "You asked me to get them right away because of bleeding risk."
- **A:** "His BP is 92/58 and heart rate is 108."
- **R:** "I think you need to see him—these are outside the parameters you gave me."

Benefits of SBAR

Standardization. Everyone uses the same format, reducing variability.

Completeness. The structure prompts inclusion of all relevant information.

Efficiency. Information is organized logically, saving time.

Assertiveness. The recommendation component encourages nurses to advocate for their patients.

Improved Outcomes. Research has shown that SBAR implementation reduces adverse events and improves team communication.

6.5 Following Up After Delegation

Delegation does not end when you give instructions. Appropriate follow-up is essential for patient safety and delegatee development. Follow-up includes verification, evaluation, and feedback.

Verification

Verify that the task was completed and the results are as expected.

Check completion. Did the delegatee actually do what you asked? Don't assume—verify.

- Review documentation
- Ask the delegatee directly
- Observe the patient if appropriate

Review results. What were the findings? Do they require any action?

- Are vital signs within expected parameters?
- Does the patient have any new concerns?
- Is follow-up intervention needed?

Identify discrepancies. If the task was not completed or results are unexpected, investigate why.

Evaluation

Evaluate both the outcome and the process.

Patient outcome. Is the patient's condition as expected? Were there any problems?

Task performance. Was the task performed correctly and completely? Was the timeline followed?

Communication. Did the delegatee report back appropriately? Were your instructions clear?

Delegation decision. Was this the right task to delegate? The right person? The right circumstances?

Use evaluation to improve future delegation decisions.

Providing Feedback

Feedback is essential for delegatee development and team function.

Positive feedback. When things go well, say so. Recognition reinforces good performance.

- "Thank you for getting those vitals quickly and reporting back right away."
- "I noticed you communicated really clearly when you told me about Mrs. Johnson's change—that was exactly what I needed."

Constructive feedback. When improvement is needed, provide feedback that is specific, timely, and focused on behavior rather than personality.

- *Poor:* "You need to be more careful."
- *Better:* "When you obtained Mr. Smith's blood pressure, the reading seemed unusually low. Let me show you how to verify accuracy by repositioning the cuff and repeating the measurement."

Timely feedback. Provide feedback as close to the event as possible while details are fresh.

Private feedback. Constructive feedback should be given privately, not in front of patients or other staff.

Two-way dialogue. Invite the delegatee to share their perspective. There may be information you don't have.

When the Delegatee Reports a Problem

When a delegatee reports abnormal findings or concerns:

1. **Thank them for reporting.** Reinforce the behavior you want.

2. **Get the details.** Use SBAR or other structured format.

3. **Assess the situation.** Go see the patient if needed.

4. **Take appropriate action.** Intervene as needed.

5. **Close the loop.** Let the delegatee know what happened and what you did.

Example: "Thank you for telling me about Mr. Chen's low blood pressure right away. I assessed him and called the physician. We're giving him a fluid bolus. You did exactly the right thing by reporting immediately."

6.6 When Things Go Wrong

Despite best efforts, problems will sometimes occur. How you respond to errors, near-misses, and adverse events matters for patient safety, team function, and professional development.

Types of Problems

Errors. Something was done incorrectly. The task was performed, but not as intended or not correctly.

Omissions. Something was not done at all. The task was skipped or forgotten.

Near-misses. Something almost went wrong but was caught before causing harm.

Adverse events. Something went wrong and the patient was harmed.

Immediate Response

When you discover a problem:

1. Ensure patient safety first. Whatever went wrong, make sure the patient is safe now. Assess, intervene, and stabilize as needed.

2. Gather information. What happened? When? What was the intended action vs. actual action? What is the current patient status?

3. Notify appropriate parties. Depending on the situation, this may include the physician, charge nurse, supervisor, and/or risk management.

4. Document objectively. Record what happened, what you observed, what actions were taken, and patient status. Document facts, not opinions or blame.

Having Difficult Conversations

After ensuring patient safety, you will need to discuss what happened with the delegatee. This can be uncomfortable but is essential.

Focus on facts and learning, not blame. The goal is to understand what happened and prevent recurrence, not to punish.

- *Blaming:* "How could you forget to check his blood sugar? That was careless."
- *Learning-focused:* "Let's talk about what happened with Mr. Jones's glucose check. Walk me through your afternoon—I want to understand the situation."

Use a private setting. Never critique a colleague in front of others.

Listen to understand. There may be system factors you are not aware of—interruptions, unclear instructions, competing demands.

Identify contributing factors. Errors are rarely caused by a single person being "bad." Usually there are multiple contributing factors:

- Communication breakdown
- System issues (staffing, resources, equipment)
- Knowledge deficit
- Process problems
- Environmental factors

Focus on improvement. What will we do differently next time? How can we prevent this from recurring?

System Thinking

Most errors in healthcare are not caused by individual negligence but by system failures. A "just culture" recognizes that:

- **Human error** is inevitable and should be addressed through system improvements
- **At-risk behavior** (taking shortcuts, workarounds) requires coaching and removal of incentives for risky behavior
- **Reckless behavior** (conscious disregard for substantial risk) requires accountability

When things go wrong, ask: "What can we change in the system to make it harder for this to happen again?"

Reporting and Documentation

Depending on the situation, various reports may be required:

Incident reports. Most facilities require incident reports for errors, near-misses, and adverse events. These reports are used for quality improvement and risk management. Complete them factually and objectively.

Communication to leadership. Notify your charge nurse and/or supervisor about significant events.

Documentation in the medical record. Document what happened to the patient, what assessment was done, what interventions were performed, and the patient's response. Do not document that an incident report was filed.

Supporting Each Other

Errors are distressing for everyone involved—the patient, the delegatee, and you. Healthcare workers experiencing "second victim" phenomenon may feel guilt, anxiety, and self-doubt after being involved in an error.

Support the delegatee. While accountability is important, so is support. A punitive response will not prevent future errors and may discourage reporting.

Seek support for yourself. If you are involved in an error or adverse event, you may also need support. Talk to a trusted colleague, supervisor, or employee assistance program.

Learn and move forward. The goal is not to dwell on what went wrong but to learn from it and continue providing excellent care.

6.7 Key Takeaways

- **Supervision exists on a continuum** from direct to indirect to available. Select the level based on task complexity, patient stability, and delegatee competency.
- **Effective delegation communication** includes the specific task, specific patient, timeline, expected findings, reportable conditions, when to report back, and opportunity for questions.
- **Closed-loop communication** (message → repeat back → confirm) reduces miscommunication.
- **SBAR (Situation, Background, Assessment, Recommendation)** provides a structured framework for clear, complete clinical communication.
- **Follow-up is essential**—verify completion, evaluate outcomes, and provide feedback.
- **When things go wrong**, ensure patient safety first, gather information, notify appropriate parties, document objectively, and focus on learning rather than blame.

6.8 Practice Problems

Directions: Select the best answer for each question. Answers and rationales are provided in the Answer Key.

1. A nurse is delegating vital signs to a UAP who has worked on the unit for five years and has demonstrated competency. The patient is stable. Which level of supervision is most appropriate?

A. Direct supervision—observe the UAP taking vital signs

B. Indirect supervision—available for questions, follow up on results

C. No supervision needed for experienced UAPs

D. Supervision is only required for new employees

2. Which delegation communication includes all essential elements?

A. "Check on 304 and let me know if there are any problems."

B. "Get vital signs on Mrs. Park in 304. Her BP has been 140s/80s. Report immediately if below 100 or above 160 systolic. I need results in 20 minutes. Questions?"

C. "Vital signs on 304 when you get a chance."

D. "Mrs. Park needs her vitals done."

3. A nurse delegates a task to a UAP. The UAP repeats back the instructions to confirm understanding. This technique is called:

A. SBAR communication

B. Closed-loop communication

C. Two-challenge rule

D. Chain of command

4. Using SBAR, which component includes "I think the patient may be developing sepsis"?

A. Situation

B. Background

C. Assessment

D. Recommendation

5. A nurse is orienting a new UAP to the unit. The UAP will perform blood glucose monitoring for the first time. Which level of supervision is required?

A. Direct supervision—observe the task being performed

B. Indirect supervision—be available for questions

C. Available supervision—can be reached by phone

D. No supervision—UAPs are trained in nursing school

6. A UAP reports vital signs to the RN: "BP is kind of low." What is the best response?

A. "Thanks, I'll check on the patient later."

B. "What are the actual numbers? I need specific values to assess the patient."

C. "You should know whether it's too low."

D. "Just document it and move on."

7. Which statement represents the "R" (Recommendation) in SBAR?

A. "Mr. Jones is having chest pain."

B. "He has a history of coronary artery disease."

C. "His vital signs are BP 168/98, HR 110."

D. "I think he needs an EKG. Can you evaluate him now?"

8. A nurse delegated vital signs to a UAP one hour ago and has not received a report. What should the nurse do?

A. Assume the vital signs were normal since the UAP didn't report

B. Wait for the UAP to report—following up seems like micromanaging

C. Find the UAP and ask about the vital signs—follow-up is part of supervision

D. Document that the UAP failed to complete the task

9. A UAP reports that a patient's blood pressure is 82/54. The nurse thanks the UAP, assesses the patient, and notifies the physician. What should the nurse do next regarding the UAP?

A. Nothing—the situation is handled

B. Criticize the UAP for not recognizing the emergency

C. Close the loop—tell the UAP what happened and acknowledge their appropriate reporting

D. File an incident report about the UAP

10. When should a nurse provide constructive feedback to a delegatee about a performance issue?

A. In front of other staff so everyone can learn

B. During the next annual performance review

C. Privately and as close to the event as possible

D. Only if the error caused patient harm

11. A nurse delegates a task but the UAP seems hesitant and asks several questions. What should the nurse do?

A. Insist the UAP perform the task—they need to learn confidence

B. Take over the task since the UAP is obviously incompetent

C. Explore the hesitation—the UAP may have a valid concern or need additional support

D. Report the UAP for insubordination

12. A medication error occurs involving a task delegated to an LPN. What is the nurse's first priority?

A. Document the error in the medical record

B. Complete an incident report

C. Ensure patient safety and assess for harm

D. Notify risk management

13. Which represents appropriate documentation after an error?

A. "LPN gave wrong dose due to carelessness. Incident report filed."

B. "Patient received 10mg instead of ordered 5mg. Physician notified. Patient assessed—vital signs stable. Continued monitoring per physician orders."

C. "Error made by LPN who should have known better."

D. "Medication error. See incident report for details."

14. A nurse overhears a UAP telling a patient, "Your blood pressure is really high—you might have a stroke!" What should the nurse do?

A. Nothing—the UAP is just being honest

B. Address this privately with the UAP—interpreting findings and providing health information is outside UAP scope

C. Report the UAP to the Board of Nursing

D. Agree with the UAP's assessment

15. Which factor would require increasing the level of supervision for a task?

A. The delegatee has performed this task many times successfully

B. The patient's condition has become unstable

C. The task is routine with predictable outcomes

D. The delegatee expresses confidence about the task

16. A nurse uses the phrase "Do you have any questions?" at the end of delegation instructions. This is an example of:

A. Closed-loop communication

B. SBAR format

C. Providing opportunity for clarification

D. Two-challenge rule

17. The "two-challenge rule" suggests that:

A. Delegates should be challenged twice before accepting a task

B. Concerns should be stated at least twice if initially dismissed

C. Two nurses should always verify critical tasks

D. Supervision should be provided by two people

18. A UAP did not complete a delegated task. After ensuring patient safety, the nurse discusses this with the UAP and learns there were multiple interruptions and competing demands. This conversation reflects:

A. Making excuses for poor performance

B. System thinking—identifying contributing factors beyond individual error

C. Avoiding accountability

D. Inappropriate supervision

19. Which is the best example of constructive feedback?

A. "You're too slow with vital signs."

B. "When you took the blood pressure, I noticed the cuff was positioned over the patient's sleeve. Let me show you the correct placement for accurate readings."

C. "You need to try harder."

D. "Everyone makes mistakes."

20. What is the primary purpose of following up after delegation?

A. To catch delegatees making mistakes

B. To ensure patient safety and evaluate outcomes

C. To demonstrate authority over team members

D. To find reasons to write up staff members

End of Chapter 6 Practice Problems

CHAPTER 7

Applying Prioritization & Delegation in Clinical Scenarios

7.1 Learning Objectives

By the end of this chapter, you will be able to:

- Apply a systematic approach to prioritization and delegation decisions
- Integrate multiple frameworks when analyzing complex clinical scenarios
- Demonstrate effective time management strategies for nursing practice
- Analyze case studies using prioritization and delegation principles

7.2 A Systematic Approach

Throughout this workbook, you have learned individual concepts: prioritization frameworks, delegation principles, scope of practice, safe assignments, and communication techniques. In real clinical practice, you must integrate all of these simultaneously. This chapter provides a systematic approach for doing so.

The PRIOD Method

When facing complex clinical situations, use the PRIOD method to organize your thinking:

P – Prioritize patients and problems

- Which patient is most unstable or at highest risk?
- Apply ABCs for emergencies, Maslow for non-emergent situations
- Consider acute vs. chronic, actual vs. potential
- Identify what must be done NOW vs. what can wait

R – Review resources

- What staff are available? (RN, LPN, UAP)
- What are their competencies and current workloads?
- What other resources exist? (charge nurse, rapid response, providers)

I – Identify delegable tasks

- Which tasks can be delegated based on scope and circumstance?
- Which tasks must you perform yourself?
- Apply the Five Rights of Delegation

O – Organize and communicate

- Give clear, complete delegation instructions
- Use SBAR for clinical communication
- Establish timelines and reporting expectations

D – Do, monitor, and evaluate

- Perform tasks you cannot delegate
- Supervise delegated tasks appropriately
- Follow up, evaluate outcomes, adjust as needed

Applying PRIOD: A Walkthrough

Scenario: You are an RN beginning your shift with four patients. During report, you learn:

- Room 401: Post-op day 1, stable, needs dressing change and ambulation
- Room 402: New admission from ED with chest pain, awaiting cardiac workup
- Room 403: Diabetic with blood glucose 52, appears diaphoretic and confused
- Room 404: CHF patient with baseline dyspnea, requesting pain medication

Your team includes yourself (RN), one LPN, and one UAP.

P – Prioritize:

- Room 403 is highest priority—hypoglycemia with neurological symptoms is an emergency (ABCs: altered perfusion to brain)
- Room 402 is second—chest pain requires assessment, but patient is awaiting workup (not actively deteriorating based on report)
- Room 404 is third—pain is actual problem but patient is at baseline
- Room 401 is fourth—stable, routine post-op care

R – Review resources:

- You (RN): Can perform all nursing functions
- LPN: Can administer medications, perform focused assessments on stable patients
- UAP: Can obtain vital signs, assist with ADLs, ambulation

I – Identify delegable tasks:

- Room 403: You must assess and treat—cannot delegate emergency care
- Room 402: Initial assessment is yours; UAP can get vital signs after you assess
- Room 404: LPN can administer pain medication after you do quick assessment
- Room 401: LPN can do dressing change; UAP can assist with ambulation

O – Organize and communicate:

- To LPN: "After I stabilize 403, please give the pain medication to Mrs. Davis in 404—she's requesting her scheduled dose. Then do the dressing change on Mr. Thompson in 401. His incision has been clean and dry. Report any redness, drainage, or dehiscence immediately."
- To UAP: "I need vital signs on the new chest pain patient in 402 as soon as I finish with my emergency in 403. His BP has been 150s/90s. Report immediately if BP above 180 or below 100, HR above 110 or below 50. Then assist Mr. Thompson in 401 with ambulation—he's steady with a walker."

D – Do, monitor, evaluate:

- Go immediately to 403, treat hypoglycemia, reassess
- Assess 402 yourself after stabilizing 403
- Check on delegated tasks, verify completion, evaluate outcomes

7.3 Time Management Strategies

Effective prioritization requires effective time management. Even perfect prioritization fails if you cannot execute your plan efficiently.

Beginning of Shift Organization

Review and prioritize during report. Don't wait until report ends to start thinking. As you receive information, begin mentally categorizing:

- Who needs immediate assessment?
- What time-sensitive tasks exist? (scheduled medications, procedures, discharges)
- What can be delegated?

Conduct quick rounds after report. Before diving into tasks, briefly lay eyes on each patient. This 5-10 minute investment often reveals urgent issues not captured in report and helps you validate your priorities.

Create a shift worksheet. Whether paper or electronic, organize your day:

- List patients with key information
- Note time-sensitive items (medications due, procedures scheduled)
- Track delegated tasks and their status
- Leave space for additions as the shift progresses

Clustering and Batching

Cluster care geographically. When possible, complete multiple tasks in the same area before moving on. If you're going to Room 401, consider what else you can do in that room or nearby.

Batch similar tasks. Medication passes, documentation, and rounding can often be done more efficiently in batches rather than scattered throughout the shift.

But never let clustering override priority. An unstable patient across the unit takes priority over convenience.

Managing Interruptions

Interruptions are inevitable in nursing. The key is managing them without losing track of priorities.

Acknowledge and triage interruptions. When interrupted, quickly assess: Is this more urgent than what I'm doing? If yes, respond. If no, note it and return to your current task.

Use the "write it down" technique. When interrupted with a non-urgent item, write it down immediately so you don't forget, then return to your task.

Communicate your plan. Let team members know what you're doing: "I'm assessing Mr. Chen right now. I'll be available in about 10 minutes." This reduces unnecessary interruptions.

Protect critical tasks. Some tasks require uninterrupted focus—medication administration, for example. Communicate this: "I'm in the middle of a medication pass. Unless it's an emergency, I'll find you when I'm done."

When You're Falling Behind

Despite best efforts, sometimes the workload exceeds capacity. When this happens:

Reprioritize. What absolutely must happen? What can wait? What can be delegated that you were planning to do yourself?

Communicate early. Don't wait until you're drowning. Tell the charge nurse: "I'm concerned I won't be able to complete Mrs. Johnson's discharge teaching before she leaves at 2pm. I need help."

Document delays. If care is delayed due to workload, document objectively: "Pain medication administered at 1045 (requested at 0930) due to competing patient care priorities."

Avoid shortcuts that compromise safety. Being behind is never justification for skipping hand hygiene, medication double-checks, or proper patient identification.

End of Shift Wrap-Up

Allow time for documentation and handoff. Don't schedule intensive tasks for the last hour of your shift. You need time to document, follow up on pending items, and prepare thorough handoff.

Complete or clearly hand off pending items. Anything not completed must be clearly communicated to the oncoming nurse.

Reflect briefly. What went well? What could improve? Brief reflection builds prioritization skills over time.

7.4 Integrating Multiple Frameworks

Real clinical situations rarely fit neatly into a single framework. Effective nurses integrate multiple frameworks simultaneously.

Framework Selection Guide

Situation	Primary Framework	Supporting Considerations
Life-threatening emergency	ABCs	--
Multiple patients, non-emergent	Maslow's Hierarchy	Acute vs. chronic, actual vs. potential
Deciding what to delegate	Five Rights	Scope of practice
Comparing problems in one patient	Acute vs. chronic, Actual vs. potential	Maslow for context
Communicating about patient	SBAR	--
Complex clinical decision	Clinical Judgment Model	All frameworks as applicable

Integration Example

Scenario: You have three patients:

- Patient A: Chronic pain patient requesting scheduled medication, also mentions new tingling in left arm
- Patient B: Post-stroke patient, stable, family asking questions about discharge
- Patient C: COPD patient with O2 sat 89% (baseline 88-90%), anxious about upcoming procedure

Integrated analysis:

Patient A initially seems low priority (chronic pain, scheduled medication). But "new tingling in left arm" is a potential acute problem that could indicate cardiac or neurological issue. **Actual vs. potential:** The chronic pain is actual but the tingling could represent an emerging emergency. **Acute vs. chronic:** New symptom in a patient with pain—could this be cardiac? This patient needs assessment before the "routine" medication.

Patient B has psychosocial needs (family questions, discharge planning). **Maslow:** These are higher-level needs (love/belonging, esteem). Patient is stable. This can wait until more urgent needs are addressed, though should not be ignored.

Patient C appears to have a breathing concern, but **change from baseline** tells us 89% is normal for this patient. However, anxiety about the procedure is an actual problem affecting the patient now. **Maslow:** Anxiety is a safety/security need that should be addressed.

Prioritization:

1. Patient A—assess the new arm tingling immediately (potential acute, possible emergency)

2. Patient C—address anxiety, provide reassurance (actual problem, safety need)

3. Patient A—administer pain medication after ruling out acute issue

4. Patient B—address family questions about discharge (stable, higher-level needs)

The "What If" Habit

Expert nurses constantly ask "what if" as they process information:

- What if this symptom is the beginning of something serious?
- What if this patient's condition changes while I'm with another patient?
- What if the delegatee encounters a problem?
- What if my assessment is wrong?

This mental habit helps anticipate problems and builds safety margins into your planning.

7.5 Case Studies

The following case studies require you to integrate multiple concepts. Work through each systematically using the PRIOD method.

Case Study 1: Medical-Surgical Unit

Setting: Day shift on a 30-bed medical-surgical unit. You are assigned four patients. Your team includes you (RN), one LPN (Maria, experienced), and one UAP (James, new to the unit but trained).

Your patients:

Mr. Adams, Room 310 — 72-year-old, post-op day 2 from colon resection

- Vital signs stable overnight
- Complaining of incisional pain 5/10
- Has not had a bowel movement since surgery
- IV antibiotics due at 0900
- Needs to ambulate twice today per orders

Mrs. Baker, Room 312 — 65-year-old admitted yesterday with pneumonia

- O2 sat 93% on 2L NC (was 91% yesterday)
- Temperature 101.2°F this morning (was 102.8°F yesterday)
- Productive cough, taking oral antibiotics
- Scheduled for chest X-ray at 1000
- Family member present asking questions about prognosis

Mr. Chen, Room 314 — 58-year-old with new-onset atrial fibrillation

- Currently on telemetry, rate controlled at 78-88
- Started on anticoagulation yesterday
- Scheduled for echocardiogram at 1100
- Anxious about diagnosis, asking many questions

Mrs. Davis, Room 316 — 81-year-old with UTI, also has dementia

- Baseline confusion but appears more confused this morning per night nurse
- Low-grade fever (99.8°F)
- On IV antibiotics, due at 0800
- Fall risk, bed alarm in place
- Family not present, lives in assisted living facility

It is now 0730. Using PRIOD, how would you organize your shift?

Consider:

- Which patient do you assess first and why?
- What can be delegated to Maria (LPN)? To James (UAP)?
- What specific instructions would you give?
- How would you communicate with the team?

Case Study 2: Priority Shift

Setting: You have organized your morning based on Case Study 1. It is now 0845. You have assessed all patients and made the following delegations:

- Maria (LPN) is giving Mr. Adams his IV antibiotic and will give Mrs. Davis hers next
- James (UAP) just obtained vital signs on all patients and is about to help Mr. Adams ambulate

Suddenly, James approaches you:

"I just checked on Mrs. Baker in 312 and she looks different. She's not talking as much and seems to be breathing faster. I got her vital signs: BP 88/52, heart rate 112, respiratory rate 28, O2 sat 88% on 2L, temp 102.4°F."

What do you do?

Consider:

- How do your priorities shift?
- What actions do you take and in what order?
- How do you communicate with your team?
- What framework(s) guide your decisions?

Case Study 3: Delegation Decision

Setting: Same unit, later that day. Mrs. Baker has been transferred to ICU. You received a new admission: Mr. Evans, 45-year-old with cellulitis of the right leg, admitted for IV antibiotics. He is stable with no significant medical history.

Maria (LPN) approaches you: "I can take the new admission if you want. I know you've had a rough morning."

How do you respond?

Consider:

- Can Maria perform the admission assessment?
- What parts of admission can be delegated vs. must be done by you?
- How do you respond professionally while maintaining appropriate scope?

Case Study 4: Ethical Considerations

Setting: End of your shift. You are giving report to the night nurse about Mr. Chen (atrial fibrillation patient). During your shift, Mr. Chen expressed significant anxiety and asked many questions. You spent extra time with him providing education and emotional support.

The night nurse interrupts: "I don't need all that detail. Just tell me if anything changed medically."

How do you handle this?

Consider:

- What information is essential to hand off?
- How do you advocate for the patient's psychosocial needs?
- How do you communicate professionally with a colleague who seems rushed?

7.6 Common Pitfalls to Avoid

As you develop your prioritization and delegation skills, be aware of these common pitfalls:

Prioritization Pitfalls

Task-focused rather than patient-focused thinking. Don't think "I need to give medications" — think "Which patient needs me most right now?"

Rigid adherence to initial plan. Your plan should be a starting point, not a straitjacket. Reprioritize constantly as conditions change.

Confusing urgency with importance. A family member demanding attention feels urgent but may be less important than the quiet patient whose condition is deteriorating.

Ignoring "soft" data. A UAP saying "something seems off" or your own gut feeling that something is wrong—these soft data points often precede hard clinical signs. Investigate them.

Anchoring on initial assessment. Just because a patient was stable an hour ago doesn't mean they're stable now. Conditions change.

Delegation Pitfalls

Under-delegating due to "I can do it faster." This is short-term thinking that leads to long-term problems. Delegate appropriately.

Over-delegating to avoid difficult tasks. Delegation should be based on scope and patient needs, not on which tasks you prefer.

Delegating without clear communication. Vague instructions lead to errors. Take time to communicate completely.

Failing to follow up. Delegation without supervision is abandonment. Always verify completion and evaluate outcomes.

Assuming competence without verification. Just because someone has a title doesn't mean they're competent for a specific task. Verify.

Communication Pitfalls

Assuming others know what you mean. Be explicit. What seems obvious to you may not be obvious to others.

Failing to close the loop. Confirm that your message was received and understood correctly.

Hierarchy inhibiting communication. Don't let position differences prevent you from speaking up about safety concerns.

Incomplete handoffs. Rushing through report leads to missing information. Take time for thorough communication.

7.7 Key Takeaways

- **Use a systematic approach** like PRIOD (Prioritize, Review resources, Identify delegable tasks, Organize and communicate, Do/monitor/evaluate) to manage complex situations.
- **Integrate multiple frameworks** simultaneously—ABCs for emergencies, Maslow for non-emergent prioritization, Five Rights for delegation, SBAR for communication.
- **Manage time effectively** through beginning-of-shift organization, clustering care, managing interruptions, and planning for end-of-shift handoff.
- **Ask "what if" constantly** to anticipate problems and build safety margins into your planning.
- **Avoid common pitfalls** including task-focused thinking, rigid plans, under- or over-delegating, vague communication, and incomplete follow-up.
- **Reprioritize continuously**—priorities shift throughout the shift as patient conditions change and new information emerges.

7.8 Practice Problems

Directions: Select the best answer for each question. Answers and rationales are provided in the Answer Key.

1. A nurse receives report on four patients. Using the PRIOD method, what should the nurse do first?

A. Identify which tasks can be delegated

B. Prioritize patients based on acuity and urgency

C. Organize the team and assign tasks

D. Review available resources

2. During morning rounds, a nurse finds: Patient A sleeping comfortably, Patient B requesting pain medication, Patient C with new-onset confusion, Patient D awaiting scheduled discharge teaching. Which patient should the nurse assess first?

A. Patient A—verify they are actually okay

B. Patient B—pain is an actual problem requiring intervention

C. Patient C—new-onset confusion could indicate serious change

D. Patient D—discharge is time-sensitive

3. A nurse has organized the morning plan but then learns a patient is returning from surgery earlier than expected. What should the nurse do?

A. Continue with the original plan—changes cause confusion

B. Reprioritize based on the new information

C. Ask the charge nurse to take the post-op patient

D. Delegate all other care to focus on the surgical patient

4. Which time management strategy is most effective at the beginning of a shift?

A. Immediately begin medication administration

B. Conduct quick rounds to lay eyes on all patients

C. Complete all documentation from the previous shift

D. Take a break to prepare mentally

5. A nurse is frequently interrupted during medication administration. Which response is most appropriate?

A. Stop what you're doing and address each interruption immediately

B. Ignore all interruptions until medications are complete

C. Acknowledge the interruption, assess urgency, and communicate your availability

D. Ask to be reassigned to fewer patients

6. A patient with chronic back pain mentions new numbness in both legs. Using integrated frameworks, this finding is:

A. Low priority because the patient has chronic pain

B. High priority because new neurological symptoms could indicate acute spinal cord problem

C. Moderate priority—address after other patients

D. Not concerning—numbness is common with back pain

7. A nurse is falling behind on tasks. Which action is most appropriate?

A. Skip documentation to save time

B. Communicate with the charge nurse and ask for assistance

C. Work faster by taking shortcuts on hand hygiene

D. Leave remaining tasks for the next shift without communication

8. An experienced UAP tells the nurse, "Mr. Jones just doesn't look right to me." The nurse should:

A. Thank the UAP but continue with planned tasks—UAPs can't assess

B. Ask the UAP to document their observation

C. Investigate immediately—"soft" data from experienced staff is valuable

D. Tell the UAP to get vital signs and report back in an hour

9. Which represents appropriate integration of frameworks for a patient with chest pain (8/10), anxiety about diagnosis, and constipation (3 days)?

A. Address constipation first—it's been present longest

B. Address anxiety first—emotional needs affect physical health

C. Address chest pain first—actual physiological problem takes priority

D. Address all three equally—they are all patient needs

10. A nurse is giving report to the oncoming shift. Which approach is best?

A. Provide only information that changed during the shift

B. Give comprehensive information including pending tasks and patient concerns

C. Keep it brief—the oncoming nurse can read the chart

D. Focus only on medical diagnoses and vital signs

11. During a busy shift, a nurse realizes that a UAP has not reported back on delegated vital signs for 45 minutes. What should the nurse do?

A. Assume the vital signs were normal

B. Wait for the UAP to report—following up might seem like micromanaging

C. Find the UAP and verify task completion—follow-up is essential

D. Document that the UAP failed to complete the assignment

12. A nurse has four patients and is trying to decide whether to cluster care geographically. Which statement is correct?

A. Always cluster care geographically for maximum efficiency

B. Geographic clustering can improve efficiency but should never override patient priority

C. Clustering care is poor practice because it delays seeing some patients

D. Only cluster care on night shift when things are slower

13. A nurse delegates vital signs to a UAP on a patient who was stable. Thirty minutes later, the patient's condition deteriorates. Who is accountable?

A. The UAP—they were responsible for the patient

B. The nurse—accountability for delegation decisions cannot be delegated

C. The charge nurse—they made the assignment

D. No one—conditions change unpredictably

14. An LPN asks the RN if she can admit a new patient to help with the workload. Which response is best?

A. "Yes, thank you—I appreciate the help"

B. "No, LPNs cannot be involved in admissions"

C. "You can help with parts of the admission, but I need to complete the initial assessment and care plan"

D. "Let me check with the charge nurse first"

15. A nurse notices a pattern: every shift, one particular task keeps getting delayed. Using system thinking, the nurse should:

A. Try harder to complete the task on time

B. Identify what system factors contribute to the delay and address root causes

C. Delegate the task to someone else

D. Accept that some delays are inevitable

16. It is 1430 and the nurse's shift ends at 1500. A patient's family arrives wanting to discuss the care plan. What should the nurse do?

A. Tell them to come back tomorrow when there's more time

B. Rush through the conversation to finish before end of shift

C. Provide what information you can, communicate the situation to the oncoming nurse for follow-up

D. Stay late to complete the conversation regardless of personal obligations

17. Using the "what if" habit, a nurse delegating vital signs to a UAP should consider:

A. What if the UAP doesn't want to do it?

B. What if the vital signs are abnormal—does the UAP know what to report?

C. What if the patient refuses?

D. All of the above

18. A nurse is caring for a patient who is stable but has a history of rapid deterioration with this condition. How should this affect prioritization?

A. No effect—prioritize based on current status only

B. This patient should be prioritized higher due to potential for rapid change

C. Delegate this patient's care so you can focus on currently unstable patients

D. Check on this patient only if time permits

19. Which scenario demonstrates task-focused rather than patient-focused thinking?

A. "Mrs. Smith's blood pressure is concerning—I need to assess her now"

B. "I need to finish my 0900 medications before doing anything else"

C. "Mr. Jones seems more confused—this could indicate a change in his condition"

D. "The new admission can wait—my current patient is unstable"

20. What is the most important principle when applying prioritization and delegation in clinical practice?

A. Efficiency—completing the most tasks in the least time

B. Patient safety—ensuring the right care is provided to the right patient at the right time

C. Fairness—distributing workload equally among staff

D. Documentation—ensuring all care is properly recorded

End of Chapter 7 Practice Problems

CHAPTER 8

Comprehensive Practice Questions

8.1 Introduction

This chapter provides comprehensive practice questions that integrate concepts from all previous chapters. These questions are designed to simulate the clinical judgment and prioritization challenges you will encounter on the NCLEX and in practice. Each question may require you to apply multiple frameworks and concepts simultaneously.

Directions: Select the best answer for each question. Answers and rationales are provided in the Answer Key.

8.2 Practice Questions

1. An RN is caring for four patients on a medical-surgical unit. Which patient should the nurse assess first?

A. A patient with COPD and O2 saturation of 89% on 2L nasal cannula (baseline 88-91%)

B. A patient one day post-appendectomy with pain rated 4/10 requesting medication

C. A patient with diabetes and a blood glucose of 68 mg/dL who is alert and oriented

D. A patient with pneumonia who was oriented earlier but is now confused and restless

2. The charge nurse is making assignments for the day shift. The staff includes one RN, one LPN, and one UAP. Which assignment is most appropriate?

A. LPN: new admission for chest pain workup; UAP: stable post-op patients

B. RN: unstable patient with sepsis; LPN: stable diabetic patients; UAP: vitals and ADLs

C. RN: patient requiring discharge teaching; LPN: patient with chest tube; UAP: all assessments

D. LPN: triage phone calls; RN: stable patients; UAP: medication administration

3. A nurse delegates vital signs to a UAP for a patient receiving a blood transfusion. Which instruction reflects appropriate delegation?

A. "Get vital signs when you have time and document them."

B. "Check vital signs every hour and let me know if anything changes."

C. "Obtain vital signs now, at 15 minutes, and at 30 minutes. Report temperature above 100.4°F, heart rate above 100, or if the patient reports chills, itching, or back pain. Find me immediately with results."

D. "The patient is stable, so just check at the end of the transfusion."

4. A nurse receives report on a patient with heart failure. The night nurse reports: "Blood pressure has been trending down from 118/72 to 98/60, urine output is 20 mL/hour for the past 3 hours, and the patient seems more tired than yesterday." Using the Clinical Judgment Model, which cognitive process should the nurse apply first?

A. Generate solutions

B. Recognize cues

C. Take action

D. Evaluate outcomes

5. An LPN reports to the RN that a patient's blood pressure is 88/52 and the patient appears pale and diaphoretic. What is the RN's priority action?

A. Ask the LPN to recheck the blood pressure in 15 minutes

B. Document the findings and notify the physician at rounds

C. Immediately assess the patient personally

D. Delegate the assessment to another RN

6. A nurse is prioritizing care for a patient who has: acute incisional pain (7/10), risk for infection related to surgical wound, anxiety about diagnosis, and a request to speak with the chaplain. Using priority frameworks, which should the nurse address first?

A. Risk for infection—prevention is always priority

B. Acute pain—actual physiological need takes priority

C. Anxiety—emotional state affects healing

D. Chaplain request—spiritual needs should not wait

7. A UAP reports to the nurse: "Mr. Thompson's blood pressure is 182/98." The nurse asks the UAP what they think is causing it. This request is:

A. Appropriate—UAPs should analyze their findings

B. Inappropriate—interpretation of findings is outside UAP scope

C. Appropriate—it develops UAP critical thinking skills

D. Inappropriate—the nurse should already know the cause

8. A nurse from a medical-surgical unit is floated to the labor and delivery unit. The nurse has no obstetric experience. Which action is most appropriate?

A. Refuse the assignment—the units are too different

B. Accept the assignment and request patients who don't require specialized OB skills

C. Accept any assignment—nursing skills are transferable

D. Call in sick to avoid an unsafe situation

9. During a busy shift, a nurse realizes that a scheduled medication is 45 minutes overdue for a stable patient. What should the nurse do?

A. Skip the dose and give the next one on time

B. Administer the medication, document the delay and reason

C. Ask another nurse to give it without explanation

D. Don't document the delay to avoid incident reports

10. A nursing student asks why experienced nurses seem to make prioritization decisions so quickly. Based on Benner's novice-to-expert theory, which response is most accurate?

A. "Experienced nurses were born with better instincts."

B. "Years of experience develop pattern recognition that allows intuitive decision-making."

C. "They're just guessing—no one really knows how to prioritize."

D. "Experienced nurses follow the same rigid frameworks you're learning."

11. A nurse is using SBAR to communicate with a physician about a deteriorating patient. Which statement represents the "A" (Assessment) component?

A. "Mrs. Garcia's blood pressure is 78/50 and her heart rate is 118."

B. "She was admitted yesterday for pneumonia and has been on IV antibiotics."

C. "I'm concerned she may be developing septic shock."

D. "I think she needs a fluid bolus and possible transfer to ICU."

12. A charge nurse notices that one RN has three high-acuity patients while another RN has five stable patients. A family member complains that it's "unfair" the first nurse has fewer patients. Which response is most appropriate?

A. "You're right—I'll redistribute the patients equally."

B. "Assignments are based on patient needs and acuity, not just numbers."

C. "That nurse is more experienced, so they should have more patients."

D. "I don't have to explain staffing decisions to families."

13. A nurse delegates ambulation to a UAP for a patient who is post-op day 1. Thirty minutes later, the nurse finds the patient still in bed. The UAP says there were "too many interruptions." Using system thinking, what should the nurse do?

A. Write up the UAP for failing to complete the assignment

B. Complete the task, then discuss what system factors contributed to the delay

C. Report the UAP to the charge nurse

D. Never delegate to this UAP again

14. According to the Five Rights of Delegation, which situation represents a violation of "Right Circumstance"?

A. Delegating vital signs to a UAP who has demonstrated competency

B. Delegating blood glucose monitoring to a UAP who was trained last week

C. Delegating vital signs on a patient who is showing signs of deterioration

D. Delegating ambulation to a UAP for a patient who walked yesterday without difficulty

15. A patient with chronic back pain suddenly reports new weakness in both legs and difficulty urinating. The nurse should recognize this as:

A. An expected finding related to chronic pain medication use

B. A low priority—chronic pain patients often have multiple complaints

C. A potential emergency requiring immediate assessment—possible cauda equina syndrome

D. A psychosomatic response to chronic pain

16. A nurse receives report that a patient is "stable" but has a "history of going bad quickly with this condition." How should this information affect prioritization?

A. No effect—base priorities on current status, not history

B. Increase this patient's priority due to potential for rapid deterioration

C. Delegate this patient's care to ensure experienced staff are available for other patients

D. Wait to see if the patient actually deteriorates before adjusting priorities

17. A UAP tells the nurse, "Something just doesn't seem right with Mrs. Johnson. I can't put my finger on it." What is the nurse's best response?

A. "That's not very helpful. What are her vital signs?"

B. "UAPs can't assess patients, so just keep doing your tasks."

C. "Thanks for letting me know. I'll go assess her right now."

D. "Document your feelings in the chart and let me know if it gets worse."

18. The RN asks the LPN to reinforce teaching about incentive spirometer use for a post-operative patient. The LPN asks, "Can't I just do the initial teaching?" What is the RN's best response?

A. "Sure, teaching is teaching—go ahead."

B. "Initial teaching requires assessment of learning needs and is an RN responsibility. You can reinforce what I've already taught."

C. "No, LPNs can't do any teaching."

D. "Ask the charge nurse for permission."

19. A nurse has completed delegating tasks to a UAP and asks, "Do you have any questions?" The UAP says no. Later, the task is done incorrectly. This situation primarily reflects a failure in:

A. The UAP's competence

B. Right Task

C. Closed-loop communication—the nurse should have had the UAP repeat back instructions

D. Right Person

20. Four patients need attention: Patient A needs scheduled medication (5 minutes late), Patient B's family has questions about discharge, Patient C just returned from surgery and hasn't been assessed, Patient D is resting comfortably with no current needs. Which patient is the priority?

A. Patient A—medications should never be late

B. Patient B—family needs are important for satisfaction

C. Patient C—post-procedure patients require immediate assessment

D. Patient D—should always check on resting patients first

21. A nurse is caring for a patient who becomes unstable. The patient had been assigned to an LPN. What should happen?

A. The LPN should continue care—they were assigned

B. The LPN should call the physician independently

C. The RN should assume care or provide direct supervision

D. The patient should be transferred to ICU immediately

22. Which task can be delegated to a UAP?

A. Evaluating a patient's response to pain medication

B. Obtaining vital signs on a stable patient with clear reporting parameters

C. Performing initial shift assessment on assigned patients

D. Deciding which patient should be seen first based on vital signs

23. A new graduate nurse is overwhelmed and afraid of making delegation errors due to being "accountable for everything." Which response from the preceptor is most helpful?

A. "You're right to be afraid—delegation is risky. Do everything yourself."

B. "Don't worry—the UAP is responsible, not you."

C. "Using the Five Rights systematically helps ensure safe delegation. It's a required part of professional nursing practice."

D. "Just delegate everything so you can focus on critical patients."

24. A patient's condition has changed, requiring the nurse to adjust the plan of care. The nurse updates the UAP: "Mrs. Chen is now on bedrest—don't ambulate her until I reassess." This is an example of:

A. Poor delegation—the nurse should ambulate the patient personally

B. Appropriate communication of changing circumstances

C. Inappropriate—UAPs don't need to know why orders change

D. Overstepping—only physicians can change activity orders

25. A nurse is giving end-of-shift report. Which approach best supports patient safety?

A. "Nothing much happened—read the chart if you need details."

B. "Comprehensive summary including status, pending items, concerns, and what to watch for."

C. "Only report things that changed—the oncoming nurse can figure out the rest."

D. "Keep it brief—detailed reports waste time."

26. Using Maslow's hierarchy, which patient need should be addressed first?

A. A patient who is anxious about a new cancer diagnosis

B. A patient who reports feeling isolated from family members

C. A patient who has moderate incisional pain 12 hours post-surgery

D. A patient who wants to discuss advance directives

27. A nurse is delegating care for four patients to an LPN and a UAP. The nurse tells the UAP, "Just help wherever needed." What is wrong with this delegation?

A. Nothing—flexibility is important in team nursing

B. The instructions lack specificity—effective delegation requires clear task assignment

C. UAPs should only help the LPN, not the RN

D. The nurse should not delegate to UAPs

28. A patient admitted for COPD exacerbation has an oxygen saturation of 91% on 2L nasal cannula. The patient says, "This is higher than my normal." How should this information affect the nurse's assessment?

A. Increase concern—if 91% is high for this patient, their baseline function is worse than typical

B. Decrease concern—the patient knows their body better than we do

C. No effect—91% is acceptable for any patient with COPD

D. Discontinue oxygen since the saturation is above the patient's normal

29. A nurse believes an assignment is unsafe but has been told there are no other options. After documenting concerns with an assignment-despite-objection form, what should the nurse do next?

A. Refuse to care for the patients and leave the unit

B. Provide the best possible care while continuing to escalate concerns

C. Care for the patients but refuse to document anything

D. Ignore safety concerns since they've been documented

30. The charge nurse receives a new admission from the ED: a patient with chest pain awaiting cardiac workup. Which staff member should receive this assignment?

A. The RN, because cardiac patients require assessment and monitoring

B. The LPN, because the patient is just "awaiting workup"

C. The UAP, because they can obtain vital signs

D. Whoever has the fewest patients, regardless of patient complexity

31. A nurse uses the PRIOD method at the beginning of the shift. After completing the "P" (Prioritize), what is the next step?

A. Identify delegable tasks

B. Do, monitor, and evaluate

C. Review available resources

D. Organize and communicate

32. A patient falls while the UAP is assisting with ambulation. The nurse's first priority is to:

A. Document the incident

B. Complete an incident report

C. Assess the patient for injury

D. Determine what the UAP did wrong

33. An experienced nurse tells a new graduate, "I never use frameworks like ABCs or Maslow—I just know what to do." According to Benner's theory, this reflects:

A. Poor practice—all nurses should use frameworks

B. Expert-level practice where pattern recognition has replaced analytical frameworks

C. Evidence that frameworks are unnecessary

D. The nurse's unwillingness to teach properly

34. A nurse is interrupted while administering medications. Another patient's family member says, "Mom's IV is beeping." What is the most appropriate response?

A. Stop immediately and go check the IV

B. Ask a colleague to check the IV while completing the medication administration safely

C. Tell the family member to wait—you'll be there when you're done

D. Ignore the interruption—medication administration is protected time

35. A UAP reports that a patient's blood pressure is "normal." What clarification should the nurse request?

A. No clarification needed—normal is sufficient

B. The actual blood pressure numbers, because "normal" is interpretation

C. Whether the UAP used proper technique

D. Why the UAP didn't report sooner

36. An RN receives report that an LPN has been caring for a patient whose condition has been stable. During rounds, the RN notes the patient is now confused with increased respiratory effort. What should the RN do?

A. Tell the LPN to continue monitoring

B. Assume care and assess the patient immediately

C. Ask the UAP to get vital signs and report back

D. Wait to see if the symptoms resolve

37. Which statement about accountability in delegation is correct?

A. Accountability transfers to whoever performs the task

B. Accountability can be shared equally between RN and delegatee

C. The RN retains accountability for delegation decisions even when responsibility is transferred

D. The facility is accountable, not individual nurses

38. A nurse is planning care for a patient with: chest pain (resolved after nitroglycerin), history of anxiety disorder, NPO for stress test tomorrow, and request for sleeping medication tonight. Using priority frameworks, which represents the correct order of priority?

A. Chest pain status, NPO status, anxiety, sleep medication

B. Anxiety, chest pain status, sleep medication, NPO status

C. Sleep medication, anxiety, NPO status, chest pain status

D. NPO status, sleep medication, chest pain status, anxiety

39. A float nurse from ICU is working on a medical-surgical unit. The charge nurse assigns the float nurse the most complex patients on the unit. This assignment is:

A. Appropriate—ICU nurses can handle complex patients

B. Inappropriate—float nurses should receive patients matching the receiving unit's typical assignment, not the most complex

C. Appropriate—it maximizes the float nurse's skills

D. Inappropriate—float nurses should not receive any patients

40. A nursing student correctly identifies that an unstable patient needs immediate assessment but hesitates because "I'm just a student." The instructor's best response is:

A. "You're right—let me handle it."

B. "Your clinical judgment is correct. Let's assess together, and you'll learn when to escalate."

C. "Students shouldn't prioritize—just follow the assignment."

D. "Ignore your instincts until you have more experience."

41. A patient admitted for pneumonia has the following findings: temperature 101.2°F, productive cough, oxygen saturation 94% on room air, and anxiety about missing work. Using Maslow's hierarchy, which finding represents the lowest (most basic) level need?

A. Anxiety about missing work

B. Productive cough

C. Temperature 101.2°F

D. Oxygen saturation 94%

42. A nurse delegates vital signs to a UAP at 0800. At 0930, the nurse realizes the UAP never reported back. What should the nurse do?

A. Assume the vital signs were normal since the UAP didn't report problems

B. Document that the UAP failed to complete the task

C. Find the UAP immediately to verify task completion—follow-up is the nurse's responsibility

D. Wait until the next scheduled vital signs

43. Which situation represents appropriate use of the "two-challenge rule"?

A. A UAP challenges the nurse's delegation twice before accepting the task

B. A nurse voices concern about a patient's deterioration; when dismissed, the nurse states the concern again more assertively

C. A physician challenges the nurse's assessment twice

D. A charge nurse challenges assignments twice before finalizing them

44. A patient with a history of opioid addiction is requesting pain medication. The nurse's first priority is:

A. Withhold medication due to addiction history

B. Assess the patient's pain, recognizing that patients with addiction history still experience real pain

C. Consult psychiatry before giving any medication

D. Give the minimum dose regardless of pain level

45. A nurse notices that documentation is consistently incomplete at shift change. Using system thinking, the nurse should:

A. Work harder to complete documentation

B. Report the previous shift nurses for incomplete documentation

C. Analyze system factors (workload, time, documentation complexity) contributing to the problem

D. Accept that incomplete documentation is inevitable

46. The nurse is preparing to call a physician about a patient with new-onset chest pain. Using SBAR, what information should be included in "Background"?

A. "The patient is having chest pain 7/10 and is diaphoretic."

B. "I think we need a stat EKG and troponin level."

C. "The patient is 67 years old, admitted for pneumonia, has a history of hypertension and diabetes, and had a cardiac stent placed two years ago."

D. "I'm calling about Mr. Roberts in room 412."

47. An RN supervises an LPN who is caring for stable patients. Which level of supervision is most appropriate?

A. Direct supervision—physically present and observing all care

B. Indirect supervision—available and accessible but not constantly present

C. No supervision needed—LPNs are licensed professionals

D. Available supervision—can be reached by phone if needed

48. A nurse is caring for a patient who becomes unresponsive. Using ABCs, what should the nurse assess first?

A. Circulation—check for a pulse

B. Airway—ensure the airway is open and patent

C. Breathing—assess for chest rise and respiratory effort

D. Call for help before any assessment

49. A patient asks the UAP, "Is my blood pressure good?" The UAP responds, "It's 142/88, which is a little high." What should the nurse do?

A. Nothing—the UAP accurately reported the numbers

B. Address this privately with the UAP—interpreting findings is outside UAP scope

C. Thank the UAP for educating the patient

D. Report the UAP to the nursing supervisor

50. Which best describes the relationship between prioritization and delegation?

A. They are separate skills that don't interact

B. Prioritization determines what needs to be done; delegation helps determine who should do it

C. Delegation is more important than prioritization

D. Prioritization only matters when you can't delegate

End of Chapter 8 Comprehensive Practice Questions

ANSWER KEY

Answer Key & Rationales

Chapter 1 Answers

1. Answer: B. Prioritization is a continuous process of reassessing and reordering patient needs. It is not a one-time decision but an ongoing cycle throughout each shift.

2. Answer: B. Effective prioritization can prevent failure to rescue by ensuring early recognition of deterioration. This is the most critical patient safety concern.

3. Answer: B. Recognize cues is the first cognitive process in the NCJMM—identifying relevant information from assessment data.

4. Answer: C. Best practice is to assess the most unstable patient first, then reassess priorities based on findings. This reflects the dynamic nature of prioritization.

5. Answer: B. According to Benner, experienced nurses develop pattern recognition over years. Frameworks help novice nurses until they develop that intuition.

6. Answer: C. Analyze cues involves considering possible reasons for findings. The nurse should analyze before taking action.

7. Answer: C. New-onset confusion could indicate serious problems such as hypoxia, infection, or stroke. This takes priority over routine tasks.

8. Answer: C. Nursing students lack the clinical experience needed for pattern recognition. This is developmentally normal, not a deficit.

9. Answer: C. Respiratory changes with low oxygen saturation and accessory muscle use require immediate reprioritization and assessment.

10. Answer: B. The NGN tests clinical judgment, which includes recognizing, analyzing, and prioritizing information.

11. Answer: C. A fallen patient must be assessed immediately for injuries. Patient safety takes priority over family discussions.

12. Answer: B. Changing the plan after learning of new chest pain demonstrates dynamic prioritization—adjusting based on new information.

13. Answer: B. For patients with COPD, an O2 sat of 90% may be acceptable. The nurse should recognize baseline varies and assess further.

14. Answer: C. Using a systematic framework helps students identify urgent needs when they cannot rely on experience or intuition.

15. Answer: B. Nurses have a professional and ethical commitment to meet each patient's most important needs. The ANA Code of Ethics addresses this.

16. Answer: B. Absent bowel sounds and pain are expected post-operative findings that require monitoring but are not emergencies.

17. Answer: D. According to Benner, quick, automatic prioritization decisions indicate expert-level practice with intuitive grasp.

18. Answer: C. The question 'Which poses greater risk to patient safety if delayed?' best guides prioritization decisions.

19. Answer: C. The statement 'stick with it no matter what' needs correction—priorities must change based on patient conditions.

20. Answer: B. Trending BP, decreased output, and fatigue together are significant cues warranting prompt assessment for possible deterioration.

Chapter 2 Answers

1. Answer: B. Using ABCs, airway is always assessed first. Without a patent airway, nothing else matters.

2. Answer: B. According to Maslow, physiological needs (pain) take priority over higher-level needs like learning or belonging.

3. Answer: C. An O2 sat of 88% is within this COPD patient's normal baseline range (89-91%). While worth monitoring, it's not an emergency.

4. Answer: C. Shortness of breath (breathing) takes priority over constipation (elimination) and chaplain visit (spiritual needs).

5. Answer: C. O2 sat of 82% represents severe hypoxemia requiring immediate intervention. This is the highest ABC priority.

6. Answer: C. Physiological and safety needs must be met before a patient can focus on higher-level learning needs.

7. Answer: B. New confusion with fever represents an acute change from baseline, possibly indicating sepsis or worsening infection.

8. Answer: B. Actual problems (current pain) take priority over potential problems (risk for infection).

9. Answer: B. ABCs are designed for emergency situations like an unresponsive patient, not routine prioritization of stable patients.

10. Answer: B. An imminent fall (potential problem with severe consequences) takes priority. Ensure safety first, then address pain.

11. Answer: B. Change from baseline means findings that differ from the patient's usual status may indicate an acute problem.

12. Answer: C. Maslow's hierarchy correctly places physiological needs before emotional needs.

13. Answer: C. Acute appendicitis is an acute, potentially life-threatening condition that takes priority over chronic conditions.

14. Answer: B. Crackles with O2 sat 91% represents a breathing concern—the highest ABC priority among these options.

15. Answer: B. Emotional needs may affect physiological needs. The nurse should recognize this connection and address both.

16. Answer: B. Being immobile with fragile skin is a risk factor (potential problem), not a current injury (actual problem).

17. Answer: C. A panic attack with hyperventilation is an acute event requiring immediate attention, unlike stable chronic conditions.

18. Answer: B. A potential problem may take priority when actual problem is minor and potential problem is imminent with severe consequences.

19. Answer: C. The unresponsive, not breathing patient has the most immediate life threat per ABCs.

20. Answer: B. Frameworks provide systematic approaches when intuition alone is insufficient. They guide, not replace, clinical judgment.

Chapter 3 Answers

1. Answer: B. Delegation transfers specific tasks requiring nursing judgment; assignment distributes overall work responsibilities.

2. Answer: B. Right Task is the first of the Five Rights—determining if the task is appropriate to delegate.

3. Answer: B. Complete delegation includes specific patient, task, timeline, parameters, and opportunity for questions.

4. Answer: C. If the UAP is not trained, the nurse should not delegate. Find a trained person or perform the task yourself.

5. Answer: C. A bed bath for a stable patient is an appropriate task to delegate to a UAP.

6. Answer: C. Both share accountability—the nurse for the delegation decision, the UAP for their own actions.

7. Answer: B. Right Circumstance considers whether the patient condition and setting are appropriate for delegation.

8. Answer: B. This is appropriate delegation with clear parameters about what to report.

9. Answer: C. The nurse remains accountable for delegation decisions. Accountability cannot be delegated.

10. Answer: B. Delegation develops team skills and improves long-term efficiency, even if initially slower.

11. Answer: C. Patient deterioration makes the circumstance inappropriate for delegation—requires RN assessment.

12. Answer: B. Nurse Practice Acts vary by state. What's permitted in one state may be prohibited in another.

13. Answer: B. First ensure patient care by completing the task, then discuss the situation with the UAP.

14. Answer: B. Right Supervision includes following up to verify completion and evaluate outcomes.

15. Answer: C. Verify training and competency before delegating—don't assume or guess.

16. Answer: C. Initial patient assessment can never be delegated—it is an RN responsibility.

17. Answer: B. When a UAP reports a patient 'seems different,' the nurse should assess promptly. This is valuable information.

18. Answer: B. 'Not trained to perform it' is a legitimate reason to refuse a delegated task.

19. Answer: C. State Nurse Practice Acts are the primary legal authority governing nursing practice and delegation.

20. Answer: C. The Five Rights provide a systematic approach to ensure safe delegation. It's part of expected professional practice.

Chapter 4 Answers

1. Answer: B. Scope of practice is determined by State NPA, Board of Nursing rules, facility policies, and individual competency.

2. Answer: B. Initial comprehensive assessment is an RN-only function that cannot be delegated.

3. Answer: B. IV push medication authority for LPNs varies by state. Check the NPA and facility policy first.

4. Answer: C. UAPs can obtain vital signs on stable patients and report findings to the nurse.

5. Answer: B. Scope of practice varies by state. Verify regulations when relocating.

6. Answer: B. LPNs work under the direction of an RN or physician—they do not practice independently.

7. Answer: C. Telling a patient the BP is 'probably nothing to worry about' is interpretation, which is outside UAP scope.

8. Answer: C. Initial education about new medications is an RN responsibility.

9. Answer: B. LPNs can administer oral medications to stable patients within their scope.

10. Answer: B. Stable post-operative patients with routine care needs are appropriate for LPN assignment.

11. Answer: C. When an LPN reports changes, the RN must assess and determine the appropriate intervention.

12. Answer: C. Interpreting whether vital signs indicate deterioration requires nursing judgment—cannot be delegated to UAP.

13. Answer: B. Scope of practice protects both patients and the nurse's license by defining legal boundaries.

14. Answer: B. When facility policy is more restrictive than state law, follow the facility policy.

15. Answer: B. Training in phlebotomy allows the UAP to perform that skill; other scope limitations remain unchanged.

16. Answer: B. LPNs can administer oral and IM medications to stable patients.

17. Answer: C. When a UAP notices a change, they should report it to a licensed nurse immediately.

18. Answer: C. The RN must personally assess and interpret findings—this is an RN responsibility.

19. Answer: C. Triage requires nursing judgment and is an RN-only function.

20. Answer: C. Check the NPA, Board rules, and facility policy before delegating to ensure it's within scope.

Chapter 5 Answers

1. Answer: B. Assignment distributes overall work responsibility; delegation transfers specific tasks.

2. Answer: C. The most important factor is matching patient acuity with nurse competency for patient safety.

3. Answer: C. Communicate limitations before accepting an assignment. The nurse lacks ventilator experience.

4. Answer: B. Accept the float but request an assignment that doesn't require specialized skills you lack.

5. Answer: B. A stable post-op day 2 patient is predictable and appropriate for a new graduate.

6. Answer: C. When a patient becomes unstable, the RN must assume care or provide direct supervision.

7. Answer: B. If concerns aren't resolved with the charge nurse, escalate through the chain of command.

8. Answer: B. The charge nurse distributing patient care at shift start is making assignments, not delegating tasks.

9. Answer: C. Float nurses should receive orientation and assignments matching their competencies.

10. Answer: B. Accept the assignment, document concerns with ADO form, and provide the best possible care.

11. Answer: B. Unequal numbers may be appropriate if the smaller group has higher acuity patients.

12. Answer: B. Lacking required competencies with no appropriate alternative assignment is a legitimate reason to refuse.

13. Answer: C. Offer assistance and notify the charge nurse about potential need for adjustment.

14. Answer: C. ADO documentation creates a record of safety concerns while meeting professional obligations.

15. Answer: A. Consider current workload and whether competencies match the new patient's needs.

16. Answer: C. Initial teaching is outside LPN scope. Notify the RN.

17. Answer: B. Float nurses should receive assignments similar to the typical workload on the receiving unit.

18. Answer: B. Once you've accepted patient responsibility, leaving without coverage constitutes abandonment.

19. Answer: C. Express concerns professionally and ask to discuss options rather than refusing outright.

20. Answer: B. Patient safety is the most important principle guiding all assignment decisions.

Chapter 6 Answers

1. Answer: B. Indirect supervision is appropriate for experienced staff performing routine tasks on stable patients.

2. Answer: B. Complete delegation communication includes specific patient, task, baseline, parameters, timeline, and opportunity for questions.

3. Answer: B. Closed-loop communication: message → repeat back → confirm understanding.

4. Answer: C. 'I think the patient may be developing sepsis' is the Assessment—your clinical judgment about what's happening.

5. Answer: A. First-time task performance requires direct supervision—physically present and observing.

6. Answer: B. Request specific values. 'Kind of low' is vague and doesn't provide actionable data.

7. Answer: D. 'I think he needs an EKG. Can you evaluate him now?' is the Recommendation.

8. Answer: C. Follow-up is part of supervision. Find the UAP and verify task completion.

9. Answer: C. Close the loop by telling the UAP what happened and acknowledging their appropriate reporting.

10. Answer: C. Provide feedback privately and as close to the event as possible for maximum learning.

11. Answer: C. Explore the hesitation—the UAP may have a valid concern or need additional support.

12. Answer: C. First priority is always patient safety—ensure the patient is safe and assess for harm.

13. Answer: B. Objective documentation of facts and actions taken. No blame or reference to incident report in chart.

14. Answer: B. Address this privately—interpreting findings and providing health information is outside UAP scope.

15. Answer: B. When patient condition becomes unstable, increase the level of supervision.

16. Answer: C. Asking 'Do you have any questions?' provides opportunity for clarification.

17. Answer: B. The two-challenge rule means concerns should be stated at least twice if initially dismissed.

18. Answer: B. System thinking identifies contributing factors beyond individual error—like multiple interruptions.

19. Answer: B. Constructive feedback is specific, behavioral, and offers correction.

20. Answer: B. The primary purpose of follow-up is to ensure patient safety and evaluate outcomes.

Chapter 7 Answers

1. Answer: B. P in PRIOD stands for Prioritize—determining which patients need attention first based on acuity.

2. Answer: C. New-onset confusion is a change from baseline that could indicate serious deterioration.

3. Answer: B. Priorities are dynamic. Reprioritize based on new information like an early surgical return.

4. Answer: B. Quick rounds after report allow you to see all patients and validate priorities.

5. Answer: C. Acknowledge interruptions, assess urgency, and communicate your availability.

6. Answer: B. New neurological symptoms (numbness in legs) in any patient requires immediate assessment—possible cauda equina syndrome.

7. Answer: B. When falling behind, communicate early with the charge nurse and ask for assistance.

8. Answer: C. 'Soft' data from experienced staff is valuable. Investigate 'doesn't look right' immediately.

9. Answer: C. Chest pain is an actual physiological problem that takes priority over psychosocial needs.

10. Answer: B. Comprehensive report including pending items ensures continuity of care.

11. Answer: C. Right Supervision requires follow-up. Find the UAP and verify task completion.

12. Answer: B. Clustering improves efficiency but should never override patient priority.

13. Answer: B. The RN retains accountability for delegation decisions—accountability cannot be delegated.

14. Answer: C. LPNs can help with parts of admission, but initial assessment and care planning are RN functions.

15. Answer: B. System thinking identifies root causes and addresses system factors, not just individual effort.

16. Answer: C. Provide what you can, then communicate to the oncoming nurse for follow-up to ensure continuity.

17. Answer: D. The 'what if' habit anticipates multiple potential problems—all of these scenarios should be considered.

18. Answer: B. History of rapid deterioration increases priority even when currently stable.

19. Answer: B. 'I need to finish my meds first' is task-focused rather than patient-focused thinking.

20. Answer: B. Patient safety—right care to right patient at right time—is always the guiding principle.

Chapter 8 Answers

1. Answer: D. New confusion in a previously oriented patient is a change from baseline indicating possible deterioration.

2. Answer: B. RN gets unstable patient, LPN gets stable patients, UAP gets vitals and ADLs—matches acuity with competency.

3. Answer: C. Complete delegation includes specific timing, parameters, symptoms to report, and urgency.

4. Answer: B. Recognize cues is the first step—identifying that these findings together are significant.

5. Answer: C. Hypotension with symptoms requires immediate RN assessment.

6. Answer: B. Acute pain is an actual physiological need that takes priority per Maslow.

7. Answer: B. Asking UAP to interpret findings is inappropriate—interpretation is outside UAP scope.

8. Answer: B. Accept the float but request patients not requiring specialized OB skills.

9. Answer: B. Administer the medication and document the delay with reason objectively.

10. Answer: B. Per Benner, years of experience develop pattern recognition that allows intuitive decisions.

11. Answer: C. 'I'm concerned she may be developing septic shock' is Assessment—your clinical judgment.

12. Answer: B. Assignments are based on patient needs and acuity, not just equal numbers.

13. Answer: B. Complete the task, then use system thinking to identify contributing factors.

14. Answer: C. Delegating vitals on a deteriorating patient violates Right Circumstance.

15. Answer: C. New leg weakness with urinary difficulty could indicate cauda equina syndrome—a potential emergency.

16. Answer: B. History of rapid deterioration increases priority even when currently stable.

17. Answer: C. 'Something doesn't seem right' from experienced staff is valuable. Investigate immediately.

18. Answer: B. Initial teaching requires assessment of learning needs—an RN responsibility. LPNs reinforce.

19. Answer: C. Closed-loop communication means having the person repeat back instructions to verify understanding.

20. Answer: C. Post-procedure patients require immediate assessment to identify complications.

21. Answer: C. Unstable patients require RN-level care. The RN must assume care or provide direct supervision.

22. Answer: B. Obtaining vitals on stable patients with clear parameters is appropriate for UAP.

23. Answer: C. Five Rights ensures safe delegation—it's required professional practice, not optional.

24. Answer: B. Updating the team about changes in patient status is appropriate communication.

25. Answer: B. Comprehensive report ensures continuity of care and patient safety.

26. Answer: C. Pain is physiological—the most basic level in Maslow's hierarchy.

27. Answer: B. 'Help wherever needed' lacks specificity. Effective delegation requires clear task assignment.

28. Answer: A. If 91% is high for this patient, their baseline function is worse than typical—increase concern.

29. Answer: B. Cannot abandon patients. Provide best care while continuing to escalate concerns.

30. Answer: A. Cardiac patients require RN assessment and monitoring skills.

31. Answer: C. PRIOD: Prioritize → Review resources → Identify delegable tasks → Organize → Do/monitor.

32. Answer: C. Patient safety first—assess for injury before documentation or investigation.

33. Answer: B. Per Benner, expert nurses have intuitive grasp without needing explicit frameworks.

34. Answer: B. Ask a colleague to check the IV while safely completing medication administration.

35. Answer: B. 'Normal' is interpretation. The nurse needs actual values to assess.

36. Answer: B. New confusion with respiratory changes requires immediate RN assessment.

37. Answer: C. RN retains accountability even when responsibility is transferred—fundamental delegation principle.

38. Answer: A. Cardiac status priority, then physiological needs (NPO), then psychosocial (anxiety).

39. Answer: B. Float nurses should receive typical unit assignments, not the most complex patients.

40. Answer: B. Validate the student's correct clinical judgment while providing supervised learning.

41. Answer: D. Oxygen saturation represents breathing/circulation—the most basic physiological need.

42. Answer: C. Follow-up is the nurse's responsibility. Find the UAP and verify completion.

43. Answer: B. Two-challenge rule: state concern; if dismissed, state it again more assertively.

44. Answer: B. All patients deserve pain assessment. Addiction history doesn't negate real pain.

45. Answer: C. System thinking analyzes workload, processes, and resources—not just individual effort.

46. Answer: C. Background provides relevant clinical history and context.

47. Answer: B. Indirect supervision—available but not constantly present—for LPNs with stable patients.

48. Answer: B. ABCs: Airway first, then Breathing, then Circulation.

49. Answer: B. Address privately—interpreting findings is outside UAP scope.

50. Answer: B. Prioritization determines what needs to be done; delegation determines who should do it.

References

American Nurses Association. (2015). Code of ethics for nurses with interpretive statements. American Nurses Association.

Benner, P. (1984). From novice to expert: Excellence and power in clinical nursing practice. Addison-Wesley.

Maslow, A. H. (1943). A theory of human motivation. Psychological Review, 50(4), 370-396.

National Council of State Boards of Nursing. (2019). Next Generation NCLEX News, Winter 2019.

National Council of State Boards of Nursing & American Nurses Association. (2019). National guidelines for nursing delegation. Journal of Nursing Regulation, 10(1), 51-59.

Made in United States
Orlando, FL
04 November 2026

90201048R00072